HANDBOOK ON
ASIAN ELEPHANTS

A compilation of basic information

Dr. Madhukar Dama
Assistant Professor

Prof. H. A. Upendra
Director

Institute of Wildlife Veterinary Research, KVAFSU,
Doddaluvara, Coorg, India - 571232

HANDBOOK ON ASIAN ELEPHANTS

A compilation of basic information

First Published: May 2014

Authors: Dr. Madhukar Dama & Prof. H. A. Upendra

Cover Page Design: Prof. H. A. Upendra

ISBN-13: 978-1499566642

ISBN-10: 1499566646

Published by The Authors on Createspace Self Publishing Platform, United States of America

To the Veterinary Profession

CONTENTS

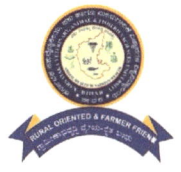

Dr. C. Renukaprasad
Hon'ble Vice-Chancellor
KVAFSU, Bidar

FOREWORD

No. VC/ROB/2013-14/182
Date: 11-01-2014

I am extremely happy to inform that IWVR, which is a constituent unit of KVAFSU, is doing a commendable service in offering PG courses in wild animal medicine and offering training program to field veterinarians.   Dr. Upendra, Director, IWVR and   Dr. Madhukar, Assistant Professor have brought out a "Hand book on Asian Elephants", a compilation of basic information on anatomical & physiological features, management, health and legal aspects of Asian Elephant. I am sure that this information will be of great help to veterinarians working in the department of AH & VS and Zoo vets in particular. As the Vice Chancellor of the university, I appreciate their effort in bringing out the information in the form of a handbook and wish them success and hope that many such useful publications will be published in IWVR.

VICE-CHANCELLOR
Vice-Chancellor,
Karnataka Veterinary,
Animal and Fisheries Sciences
University, BIDAR

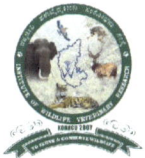

PREFACE

We are very happy to place before you "Handbook on Asian Elephants – A compilation of Basic Information", with a hope to provide all the basic information about Asian elephants in one book.

The field veterinarians working in the province of Karnataka, especially in elephant inhabited areas, expressed many a times difficulty in finding reference information on elephants. We also felt the need for the same. To address this need we planned to compile information on the Asian elephants covering various areas like its management, nutrition, health care, post-mortem, legal aspects so on and so forth. Hence, this script is presented as a handy reference which can be of help to field veterinarians, veterinary students at graduate and post-graduate degrees, researchers working with elephants, teachers of basic as well as veterinary sciences, amateurs interested to know about elephants, and anybody interested in elephants.

The structure of the book makes it very easy to read and access the required information in bulleted texts in short time. This will be of help to readers looking for specific information without loss of details. Further, pictures, illustrations, tables and diagrams placed on most of the topics will enhance the depth of the information accessed in short time.

While conducting workshops and training programs on elephants, we had tough times retrieving even basic information on Asian elephants, and felt a need for reference books, especially focused on veterinary aspects of Indian elephants, which was further echoed by request of our trainees to come up with a reference book which can be useful for field use. This motivated us to spend long hours for more than 2 months and compile this handbook.

Writing this book not only helped us compile the information in once place, but also increased our knowledge on elephants to a large extent as we browsed through numerous review articles, research articles, books, websites and conference proceedings. However, we also took care not to include unnecessary information so that this book can remain handy. Some of the resources have been a major source for compilation of this book, like i) Healthcare Management of

Captive Asian Elephants, ii) Techniques & procedure for post-mortem of elephants - A Handbook for Veterinarians, Biologists & Elephant Managers, iii) Veterinary management of captive Asian elephants and iv) Biology, medicine, and surgery of elephants. We will be indebted to the authors of these books.

We would like to thank Dr. Renukaprasad, Hon'ble Vice Chancellor, KVAFSU, Bidar; Prof. Shivaprakash, Director of Extension, KVAFSU, Bidar, and Prof. Y. Basavaraju, Former Director of Extension, KVAFSU, Bidar for their support, guidance and motivation in bringing out this work.

H. A. Upendra & Madhukar

Chapter 1

THE ASIAN ELEPHANT

Taxonomy:

Kingdom	-	Animalia
Phylum	-	Chordata
Class	-	Mammalia
Order	-	Proboscidea
Family	-	Elephantidae

Common Names: Asian Elephant, Indian Elephant

Status (Red List category): Endangered, as it is facing a very high risk of extinction in wild in the near future.

Distribution in India: from being widespread once, now the elephants of India are restricted to four regions:

1. *North-eastern India* - extends from the eastern border of Nepal in northern West Bengal through western Assam along the Himalaya foothills up to the Mishmi Hills. Towards the eastern side of the Mishmi Hills it extends into eastern Arunachal Pradesh, the plains of upper Assam, and the foothills of Nagaland. Further west, it extends to the Garo Hills of Meghalaya through the Khasi Hills, to parts of the lower Brahmaputra plains and Karbi Plateau. Isolated herds occur in Tripura, Mizoram, Manipur, and the Barak valley districts of Assam.

2. *Central India* - fragmented populations are found in Orissa, Jharkhand, and the southern part of West Bengal, and rarely in Chhattisgarh.

3. *Northwestern India* – six populations occur at the foot of the Himalayas in Uttaranchal and Uttar Pradesh, ranging from Katerniaghat Wildlife Sanctuary in Bahraich Forest Division in the east, to the Yamuna River in the west.

4. *Southern India* – occur in eight main populations mainly distributed in the hilly terrain of the Western Ghats and in parts of the Eastern Ghats across Karnataka, Kerala, Tamil Nadu, and, recently, Andhra Pradesh. The eight populations are fragmented into 1) northern Karnataka 2) the Crestline of Karnataka–Western Ghats 3) Bhadra–Malnad 4) Brahmagiri–Nilgiris–Eastern Ghats 5) Nilambur–Silent Valley–Coimbatore 6) Anamalais–Parambikulam 7) Periyar–Srivilliputhur 8) Agasthyamalais.

Habitat and Ecology: Asian elephants occur in grassland, tropical evergreen forest, semi-evergreen forest, moist deciduous forest, dry deciduous forest and dry thorn forest, in addition to cultivated and secondary forests and scrublands from sea level to over 3,000 meter above sea level

Elementary facts about the Asian elephants
➢ The Asian elephant is one of the few herbivores still existing on earth that reaches an adult body weight of more than 1000 kg.
➢ Due to their poor digestibility and size, elephants spend 14-19 hr/day feeding on large quantities of food.
➢ Elephants browse on a variety of grasses, bushes and plants based on season and habitat.
➢ Elephants defecate 16-18 times in a day discharging more than 100 kg of dung. Dung also helps disperse germinating seeds.
➢ Elephants range over large areas that may reach up to 600 km². Due to the large home range, elephants are called "umbrella species" as their conservation will also protect a many other species occurring in their habitat.
➢ As elephants have a huge ecological impact, they are regarded as a premier "flagship species" and are further considered to be a "keystone species" because of their key role in the maintenance of the ecological balance.
➢ The life span of Asian elephants is 60 to 70 years, and males reach sexual maturity between 10–15 years of age; females usually give first birth at 15 or 16 years.
➢ An elephant's eyesight is very poor and hence relies very much on its sense of smell.
➢ An elephant's trunk is formed by fusion of the upper lip and nose.

- Dog sitting posture or "sternal recumbency" in elephants is dangerous. The pleural cavity around the lungs is absent in elephants and they may die of suffocation if made to sit in the dog sitting posture for long periods.
- Elephant skull has several sinuses which make the head not as heavy as it may appear.
- Elephants are a valuable commodity and need to be handled with care and respect.
- Elephants are prone to arthritis because of the vertical position of their limbs.
- Elephants are the only living member of the order *Proboscidea*.
- Elephants can perceive sound frequencies inaudible to the human ear.
- Elephants cannot be completely domesticated.
- Elephants cannot jump up because their legs are not shaped correctly for absorbing the shock of a jump.
- Elephants drink 200- 250 liters of water a day: 50-60 liters at a time for 3-4 times a day. A trunkful can retain 6-10 liters of water.
- Elephants have a remarkable memory of events and people.
- Elephants have nails rather than hooves. Most of the elephants have 18 nails, 5 each in the front legs and 4 each in hind legs. Very rarely the total of nails goes up to 20.
- Elephants have sparse hairs (almost nude), small eyes, big head, no sweat glands, movable ears, and highly elongated upper incisors and snout that forms tusks and trunk respectively.
- Elephants travel extensively in search of food, shade and water.
- Elephants urinate 10-15 times a day with total quantity of urine about 50 – 60 liters.
- Elephants walk at a slow pace of 4km/hour and can run for a short distance up to 30 km/hr.
- In a cow elephant, the vulval opening is between the hind legs.
- Elephants have temporal gland, which secretes androgen rich dark discharge. During musth, temporal gland activity in bulls is accompanied by behavioral changes, particularly aggression, increased libido and disobedience to commands.

➢ Mammary glands are found between the forelegs. Usually cow elephants suckle their offspring for 4-5 years, but in captivity the calves are weaned after 2 years.

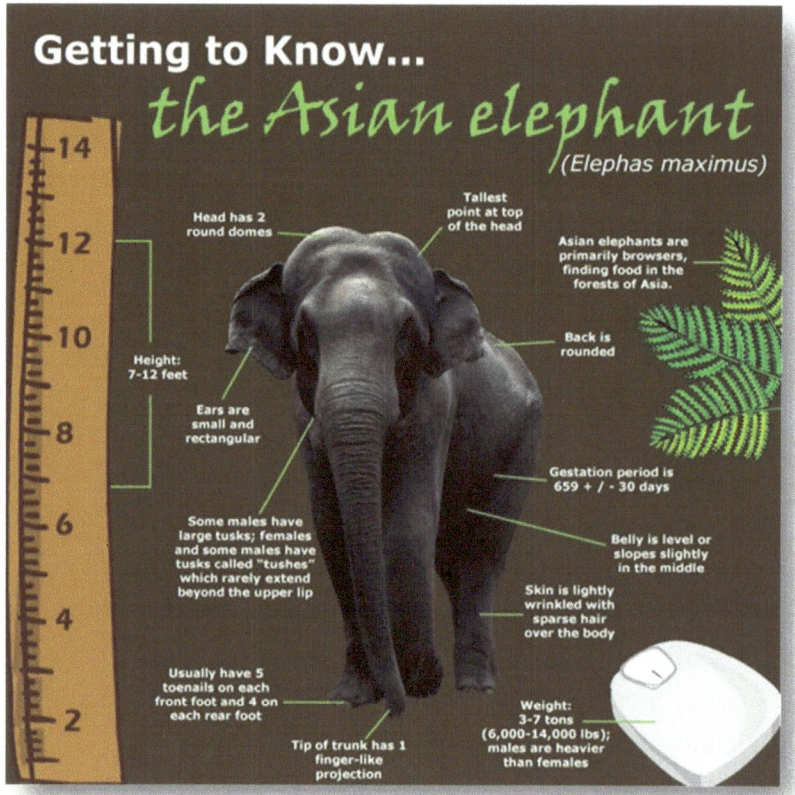

Figure 1: General features of the Asian elephant.
http://www.noahsarkzoofarm.co.uk/pages/attractions/elephant-eden/images/asian-characteristics-large.jpg

➢ Respiratory rate in elephants is 10 per minute while standing and 5 per minute during recumbency.
➢ The elephant has only two pairs of teeth, at a time and they get replaced 5 times during its lifetime.
➢ The gestation period in elephants is 21 months. Calf at birth weighs 80-100 kg and 90-100 cm in height.
➢ The heart of an elephant does not have a pointed apex and have bifid apex.
➢ The normal body temperature of the elephant is 96.6 degree F
➢ The skin is very thick and has several folds and wrinkles.

➢ The testes of a male elephant are placed abdominally.

➢ The tongue has restricted movement and cannot be protruded out.

➢ The tusk is an outgrowth or an extension of the upper incisor teeth. In males, it starts growing at 2.0 -2.5 years and grows at the rate of 3-4 inches every year.

➢ The upper ridge of the ear starts folding inwards, from the age of 10 and folds about an inch, in 20 years.

➢ There is no gall bladder in the elephant.

➢ There is no naso-lacrimal duct in elephants and hence water runs out of the eyes constantly.

➢ The African (*Loxodanta africana*) and Asian elephant (*Elephas maximus*) are the two species of elephants that differ in some features. There are three sub-species of Asian elephant (Sri Lankan, Mainland and Sumatran) and two in African elephant (Forest and Bush).

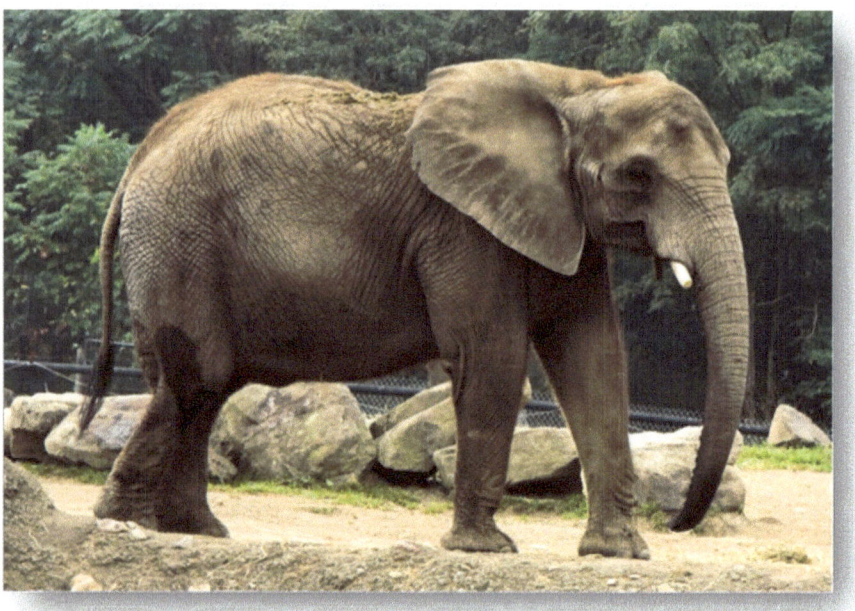

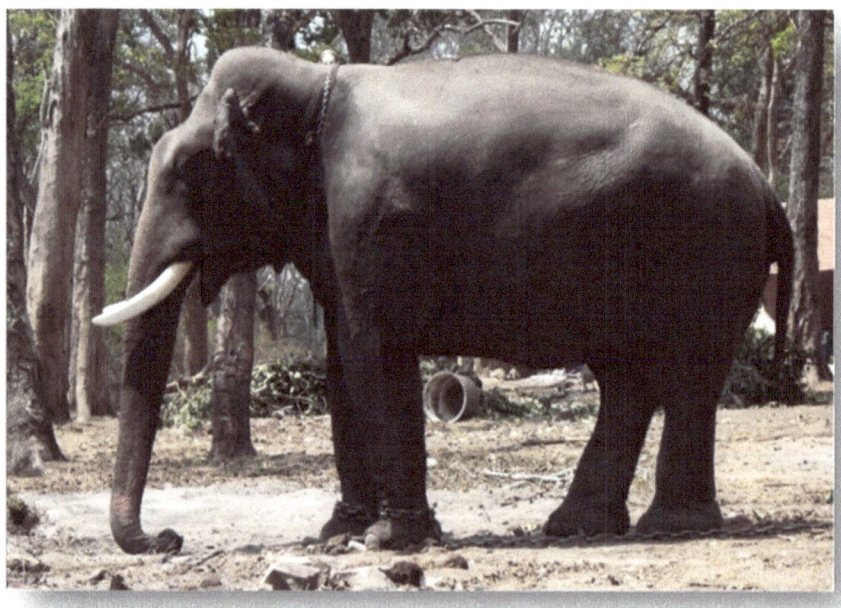

Figure 2: African elephant (top) and Asian elephant (bottom). Image of African elephant by Jason Pratt, distributed under creative commons attribution
(http://upload.wikimedia.org/wikipedia/commons/b/b1/African_Elephant_8.jpg). Image of Asian elephant by Madhukar.

Differences between Asian and African elephants		
Feature	Asian elephant	African elephant
Ears	Small	Large and covers the shoulders
Height (max, mts) – male	2.25 to 2.75	Up to 3.6
Height (max, mts) – female	2.1 to 2.4	2.3 to 2.7
Weight (max, tons) – male	3.7 to 4.5	
Weight (max, tons) – female	2.3 to 3.7	2.3 to 4.0
Tusk	Long and slender. Found only in males (Makhnas-tuskless males). Females have small rudimentary structures called tushes.	Short and stout. Found in both sexes
Trunk	Rigid with less rings, one finger at the tip and relatively longer	Flexible with more rings, two fingers at the tip and relatively short
Head	Two humped	Smooth and curved
Highest point of the body	Tip of head	Tip of shoulder
Dorsal side of the back	Convex	Concave
Ribs (Up to, pairs)	20	21
Skin	Smooth with age dependent increase in depigmentation	Coarse, loose and no depigmentation
Nails	Five on forefoot and 4 on hind foot	Four on forefoot and 3 on hind foot
Temporal gland secretion	Only in males	Both sexes
Molar laminae	Elliptical	Semi-lunar

Compiled from 1). Healthcare Management of Captive Asian Elephants, Eds. Ajitkumar and others, Faculty of Veterinary and Animal Sciences, Kerala Agricultural University, Kerala 2009. 2). Ajithkumar Santra. Handbook on wild and zoo animals. International book distributing company. 2008.

Chapter 2

ANATOMICAL AND PHYSIOLOGICAL FEATURES OF THE ASIAN ELEPHANT

Elephants resemble any other mammal anatomically and physiologically, with some exceptions related to the trunk, tusks, respiratory and reproductive systems.

Skeletal system

The skeleton is large and heavy and weighs approximately 16.5 percent of body weight.

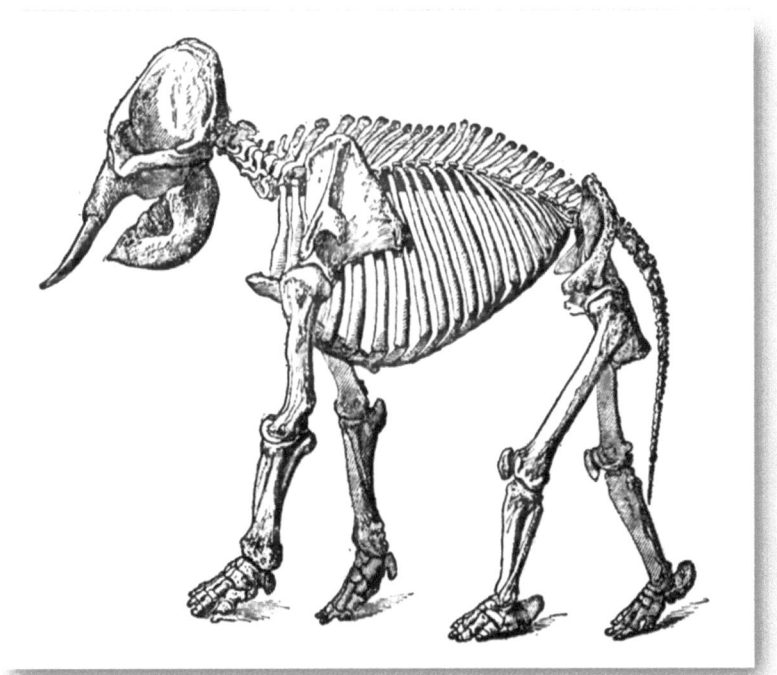

Figure 1: Skeleton of an elephant. *Image by Richard Lydekker, distributed under creative commons attribution.*
http://upload.wikimedia.org/wikipedia/commons/thumb/7/74/ElephantSkelLyd2.png/745px-ElephantSkelLyd2.png

Skull
- ➢ The skull is large and light due to numerous honey comb like air compartments.
- ➢ Pneumatization of the skull bones occurs at 3-4 years of age.
- ➢ Large skull supports attachment of trunk in addition to the usual functions like other mammals.
- ➢ Molar teeth are housed in the maxillary and mandibular bones
- ➢ Tusks are housed in the alveolar sockets of the maxillary bones.
- ➢ The skull is of similar shape in both the sexes, with skulls of young ones being dorsoventrally flattened.
- ➢ The ratio of forehead length, head length and occiput length of the skull can be used to determine the sex of the elephants.

Vertebrae
- ➢ Divided into cervical (7), thoracic (19-20), lumbar (4-5), sacral (4-5) and coccygial or caudal (24-33). The vertebral column is linearly curved and arch like.
- ➢ Vertebral junctions are tightly fixed which largely limits the movement of the vertebrae.
- ➢ Due to absence of anticlinal vertebrae, sideward bending is limited.

Ribs
- ➢ Depending on the subspecies, 19-20 pairs of ribs are found in Asian elephants in the massive ribcage that reaches up to the sternum.
- ➢ The first six pairs of ribs are sternal, the next nine pairs are asternal and last four or so pairs are true floating ribs in the Asian elephants.
- ➢ As sternum and pelvic symphisis is dorsoventrally arranged (unlike horizontal in other mammals),

elephants cannot rest on the sternum and a fall on sternum may be fatal.

➤ Inclined pelvic symphasis brings the genitals between thighs.

Limbs

➤ Limbs are strong, support heavy weight, and are placed vertically like pillars.

➤ Vertical placement (unlike angular in other mammals) limits the sideways and backward movements, which increases the chances of arthritis.

➤ Marrows are absent in the long bones, instead, haematopoeisis occurs in the dense network of cancellous tissue.

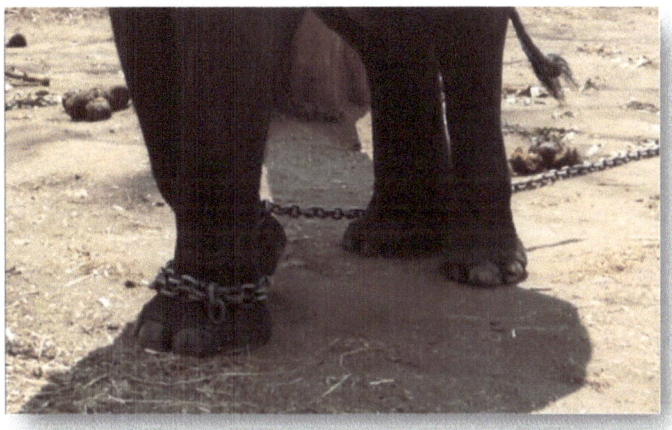

Figure 2: Asian elephant limbs. Observe the structure of nails and cushion pad. *Image by Madhukar Dama.*

➤ Replacement of marrow with cancellous structure helps the bones withstand heavy weight of elephants.

➤ The sole is made of thick and soft white elastic fibers, called cushion pad that further supports the massive weight and gait of the elephant.

➤ Elephants can walk, run and swim; however, they do not trot, canter, gallop and jump.

➢ Normally an elephant gait involves lifting two feet on one side of the body together while the two feet on the other side remain on the ground (a rack gait).
➢ Elephant walks at 4 km/hour, but can outrun humans by running at a speed of 30 km/hr.
➢ Elephants can remain standing for long periods and sleep, because of the position of bones and limbs.

Muscular system

One feature of the muscular system is large size of the muscles.

Trunk

➢ Trunk is composed of muscles, vessels, nerves, fat, connective tissues, and skin.
➢ Trunk is a fusion of the muscles of nose, upper lip and cheeks.
➢ The body of the trunk contains no bones or cartilage.
➢ Trunk is made of approximately 150,000 muscles.
➢ Superficial muscles run longitudinally along the dorsal, ventral and lateral aspects whereas internal muscles are deeply placed in radial and transverse direction.
➢ Nostrils are separated by a membranous septum and are connected to the cranium.
➢ Elephants rise and wave the trunk in the air to collect and detect the smell.
➢ Trunk is used for feeding, watering, dusting, smelling, touching, communicating (touch and sound promoter), defense and other purposes.
➢ Adult elephants can hold 10 liters of water in the trunk.
➢ The trunk also functions as a smelling organ in association with the vomeronasal organ located on the palate of the mouth.
➢ Elephants can locate female in heat over long distance and water located up to 50 km away.

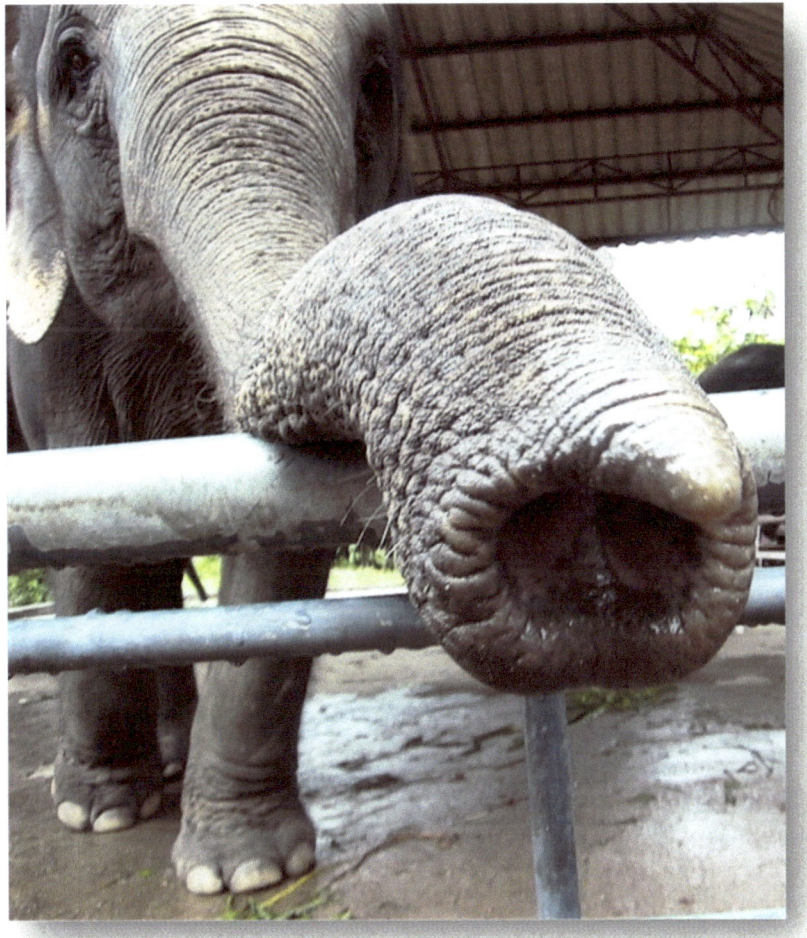

Figure 3: Trunk of an Asian elephant.
Image by Greg George, distributed under creative commons attribution.
http://upload.wikimedia.org/wikipedia/commons/thumb/c/ce/Asian_elephant_trunk.jpg/520px-
Asian_elephant_trunk.jpg

Integument system

Skin and Hair

> ➢ Elephant skin has uneven thickness, with thin skin about
> 1.8 mm found in the ear, around the mouth and anus and

thick skin of 25 to 35 mm found on the head, back and buttock.

➢ Elephant skin has a rich nerve supply and is highly sensitive.

➢ Skin is grayish and sparsely covered with hairs.

➢ With age, localized depigmentation occurs on forehead, neck, ears and forelimbs.

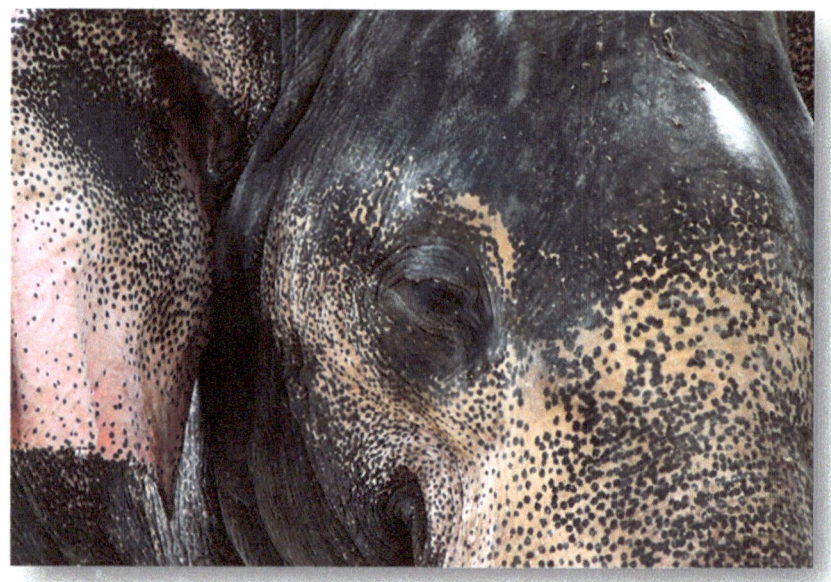

Figure 4: Depigmentation in an Asian elephant.
Image by Vinod Sivan, distributed under creative commons attribution.
http://upload.wikimedia.org/wikipedia/commons/a/a3/Elephant_-_Guruvayur.JPG

➢ Elephants keep their skin covered with soil, dust or mud, which protects them from ultraviolet radiations, dehydration and insect bites.

➢ Young elephants have hairs on the head and back.

➢ The hairs become sparse with age, mainly concentrated around eyes, mouth, chin, ear and the tip of the tail.

➢ Hairs may be brownish, brown, black, white or gray.

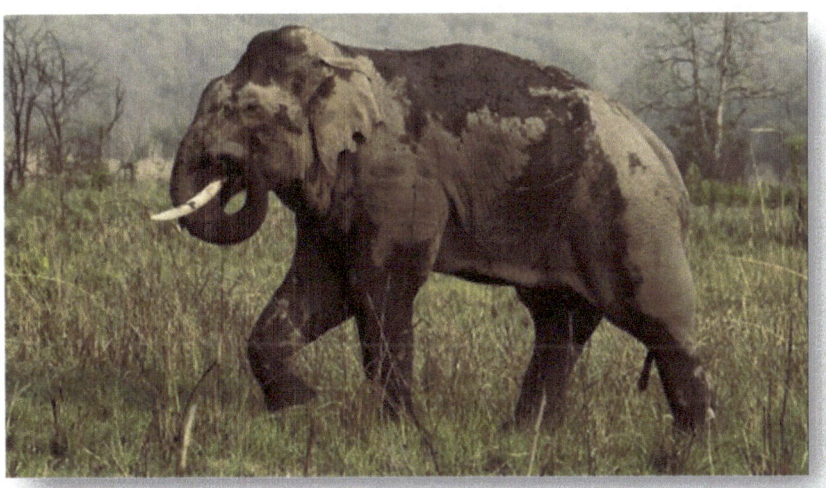

Figure 5: A mud bathed Asian elephant.
Image by Vikram Gupchup, distributed under creative commons attribution.
http://upload.wikimedia.org/wikipedia/commons/c/cd/Asian_Elephant_at_Corbett_National_Park4.jpg

Nail and plantar pad

> ➢ Elephant nails are histologically similar to other mammals.
> ➢ The nails grow about 10 mm per month.
> ➢ The keratinized sole is 4 to 12 mm thick and grows at the rate of 5 to 10 mm every month.

Sweat gland

> ➢ Elephants have very few sweat glands which are limited to the coronet line of the toenail.
> ➢ In elephants, large ears replace the conventional role of thermoregulation played by sweat glands in most other mammals.

Temporal or musth gland

- ➢ Musth gland is a large modified sebaceous gland that can be seen placed midway both the sides between eye and ear on the temple.
- ➢ The glands are covered with thick skin and produce dark, thick and foul smelling androgen rich secretion that plays important role in reproduction.

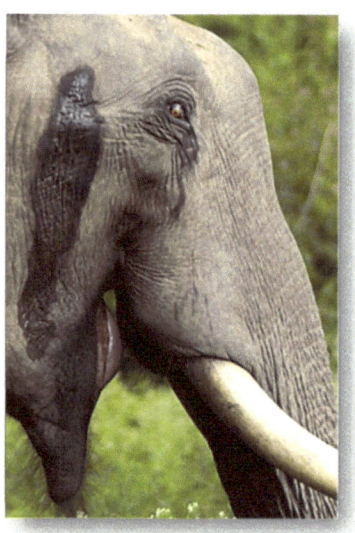

Figure 6: Temporal gland secretion in Indian elephant during musth. *Image by Yathin S Krishnappa, used under creative commons attribution. http://upload.wikimedia.org/wikipedia/commons/5/59/2005-tusker-musth-crop.jpg*

Respiratory system

- ➢ Respiratory conducting portion is formed by external nares, nasal tubes, internal nares, pharynx, larynx and trachea. The respiratory portion is formed by bronchi, bronchioles, alveolar duct and alveolar lung sac.
- ➢ Unlike other animals, the lungs are attached to the thoracic walls and diaphragm, which obliterates the pleural space normally maintained at negative pressure. Hence, elephants mostly use intercostals and diaphragmatic muscles of respiration.

> Because of this limitation, even a minor damage to the thoracic muscles and sternal recumbancy may lead to severe dyspnoea.

Gastrointestinal system

> Elephants are one of the largest monogastric herbivores.
> The digestive tract is comprised of the mouth, pharynx, esophagus, stomach, small intestine and large intestine, cecum, rectum and anus, with overall anatomy resembling to that of the horse. Accessory organs include molar teeth, tongue, salivary gland, liver and pancreas.
> Elephants do not have gall bladder and digest the food by bacterial fermentation in the cecum.
> Elephants have very poor digestive ability and they digest only less than half of the food consumed.
> Quantity of the food and water consumed by an adult Asian elephant in a day equals to approximately 10% of their body weight. This has to be increased during special circumstances.

Mouth
> Elephants have a relatively smaller mouth compared to body size.
> The oral cavity has molar teeth, a tongue, and openings of the salivary ducts and salivary glands.
> The mouth is connected to the pharynx and the upper respiratory tract.
> Elephants masticate the food by co-coordinating the movements of mandible, tongue and molar teeth.

Molar teeth
> Over a lifetime, elephants grow 2 incisors/tusks, 12 deciduous premolars and 12 molars.

> Unlike most mammals, which grow baby teeth and then replace them with a single permanent set of adult teeth, elephants have cycles of tooth rotation throughout their lives.
> The molars are replaced six times in a typical elephant's lifetime.

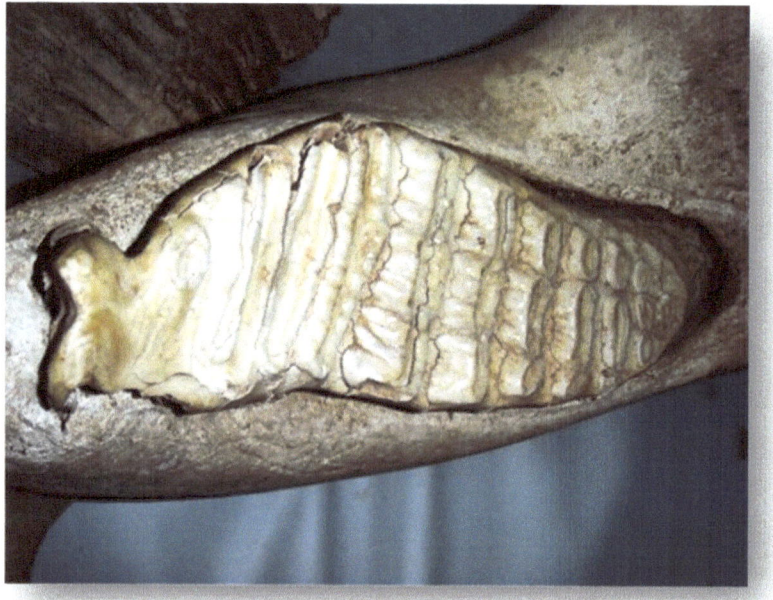

Figure 7: The molar tooth of an elephant.
Image by Challiyan, used under creative commons attribution.
http://upload.wikimedia.org/wikipedia/commons/a/a9/Elephant_teeth.jpg

> Unlike other mammals, teeth are not replaced by new ones emerging from the jaws vertically; instead, new teeth grow in at the back of the mouth and move forward to push out the old ones.
> First molars are replaced at two to three years, second molars are replaced at four to six years, and third molars are replaced at 9–15 years of age, and set four lasts until 18–28 years of age. The fifth set of teeth lasts until the elephant is in

its early 40s. The sixth (and usually final) set lasts through the rest of its life.

➢ Hence, at any given time, the elephant dental formula will be 2 (I 1/0; C0/0; PM 1/1; M 0/0) or 2 (I 1/0; C0/0; PM 0/0; M 1/1).

➢ The teeth develop before birth and newborns carry 2-3 teeth in each jaw quadrant within first few months of age.

➢ The average weight of the teeth of elephants is approximately 5 kilograms.

➢ Elephant teeth are complex like other mammalian teeth and comprise of cementum, enamel, dentin, a pulp cavity and pulp tissue that includes odontoblasts, odontocytes, vessels and nerves.

➢ The shape of projections on molar occlusal surfaces can be used to identify the elephant species. Molar projections are lozenge shaped in African elephants and loop shaped in Asian elephants.

Tusk

➢ Upper deciduous incisors are replaced at 6-12 months by the modified incisors called tusks which grow throughout the life of an elephant at about 17 cm a year.

➢ A newly developed tusk has a smooth enamel cap that eventually wears off.

➢ The dentine is known as ivory and its cross-section consists of crisscrossing line patterns, known as "engine turning", checkered pattern (a net liked pattern) which create diamond-shaped areas. This feature differs with ivory of different animals and can be used to forensically identify the specimen.

➢ As a piece of living tissue, a tusk is relatively soft; it is as hard as the mineral calcite.

➢ At least one-third of the tusk contains the pulp and some have nerves stretching to the tip.

- The tusk cannot be removed completely without harming the animal, and once removed, it has to be placed in cool and moist condition, or else it dries and cracks.
- Elephants use tusks for a variety of purposes like digging for water, salt, and roots; debarking or marking trees; and for moving trees and branches when clearing a path, to attack and defend, and to protect the trunk.
- Elephants preferentially use on tusk over another, a feature similar to handedness in humans.
- The dominant tusk worn out and become shorter and rounded at the top with age.
- Hunting for elephant ivory may progressively select for smaller tusks with future generations growing progressively smaller tusks.
- The structure of tusk is similar to that of a tooth except that enamel is only found on milk tusks.
- About 1/3rd of the tusk length lies in the alveolar socket of the maxillary bone.
- Some tuskless males, called makhnas, may be more robust than Tuskers.

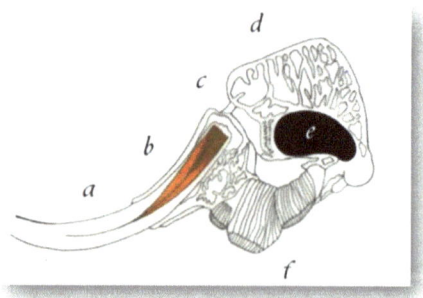

Figure 8: Longitudinal section of elephant head and tusk showing external tusk (a), pulp cavity (b), internal nare (c), air cavities (d), brain (e) and molars. *With modifications from Groning 1999.*

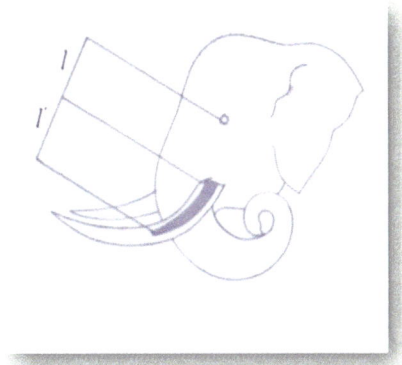

Figure 9: Estimation of the extent of pulp cavity for trimming of elephant tusk. The sulcus is approximately the length between the eye and the tusk sulcus. The pulp of the tusk extends about 2/3 of the tusk length. The position of the pulp is important for properly trimming the tusk. *With modifications from Robinsom and Schmidt, 1986.*

Esophagus
- ➤ Elephant esophagus is musculomembranous with numerous mucous glands that keeps the food lubricated during transit.

Stomach
- ➤ The elephant stomach is cylindrical.
- ➤ Adult stomach is approximately 75-90 cm long with a volume of 30 to 70 liters.

Intestine, cecum and rectum
- ➤ The small and large intestines are 65-75 feet and 35-45 feet respectively.
- ➤ The cecum, 5 to 7 feet long, is a major site of fermentation in the elephant.
- ➤ The small and large intestine can hold a volume of 135 liters and 480 liters of feed in adult elephant.

Liver and pancreas
- ➢ Elephants do not have a gall bladder.
- ➢ Multiple ducts running from liver transport bile to the small intestine.
- ➢ Pancreatic secretions facilitate protein and carbohydrate digestion in the intestine.

Circulatory, hemopoetic and lymphatic systems

Heart
- ➢ Adult elephant heart weighs 12 to 21 kgs, has a bifid apex and only one coronary artery.
- ➢ Large sinuses along the trachea, sternum, axillae, inguinal area and sides of the temporal area moderate the high blood pressure from cardiac contraction.
- ➢ The vasculature is thicker walled and stronger than other mammals.

Blood
- ➢ Except larger size of the blood cells, all the features are similar to other mammalian blood.

Lymph and lymphoid organs
- ➢ The thymus, tonsils, lymph nodes and spleen are the lymphoid organs of the elephant that play major role in elephant immune response.

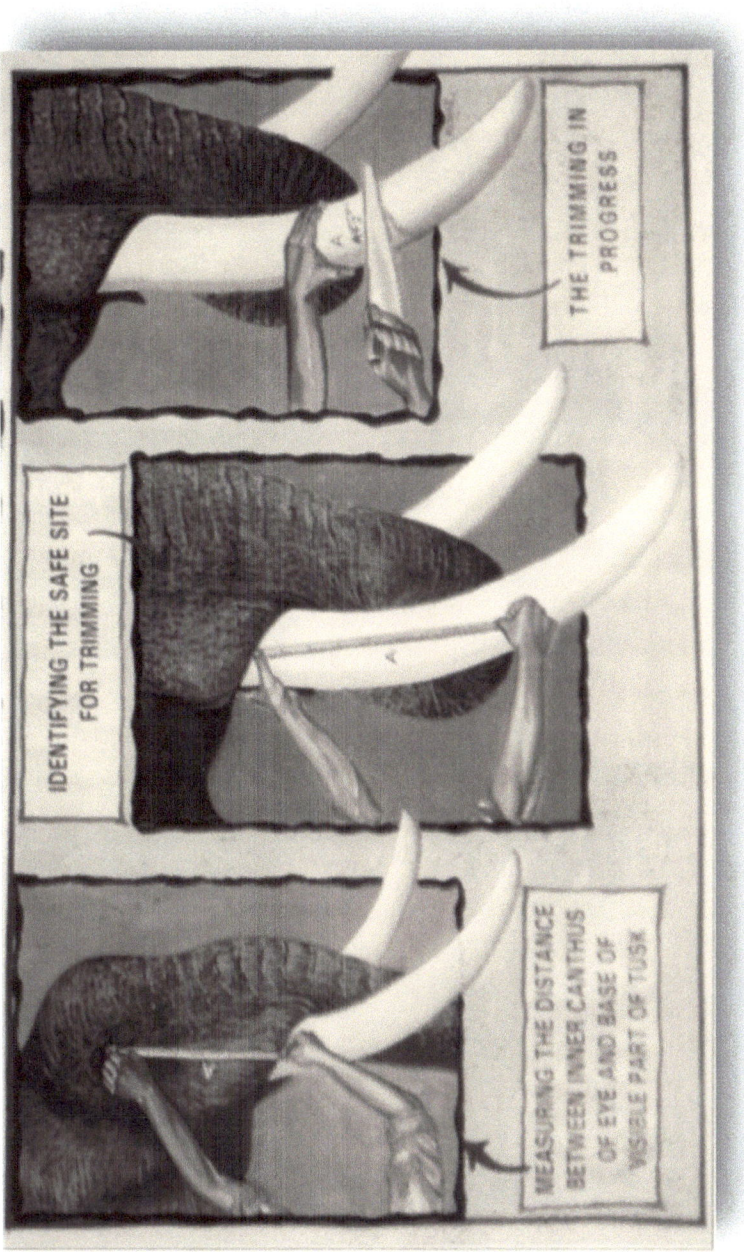

Figure 10: Estimation of safe site for trimming of elephant tusk. Measure the distance from inner canthus of the eye to the base of the trunk. Now, mark the trunk at this length from the base of the trunk, this gives the safe distance for trimming. *(Modified and adapted from Healthcare Management of Captive Asian Elephants, Eds. Ajitkumar and others, Faculty of Veterinary and Animal Sciences, Kerala Agricultural University, Kerala 2009)*

Nervous system

> Like other mammals, the nervous system is comprised of a brain, spinal cord and peripheral nerves. Interestingly, though brain to body size ratio is smaller in elephants compared to many other mammals, they are regarded as cognitively superior, mostly due to grossly large size of the brain and complex arrangements of gyri and sulci.
> Male adult brain can weigh 4.5 kg, whereas female elephants can have a 4.2 kg brain, with no difference in intelligence between sexes.
> The spinal cord of the elephant has two nerve rich enlargements, called cervical and lumbar enlargements which coordinate limb movements.

Urinary system

> Elephant kidney is multilobed, with 5-7 lobules resembling cattle kidneys.
> The adult elephant urinary bladder can hold 6-18 liters of urine.
> Elephants urinate up to 50 liters of urine in a day over 10-15 acts of urination.

Reproductive system

Male

> A male elephant's testes are located internally near the kidneys (Testiconda), and each can weigh up to 2 kgs.
> All accessory glands and features of spermatozoa are similar to most other mammals.
> The elephant's penis can reach a length of 100 cm (39 in) and a diameter of 16 cm (6 in) at the base.

- ➤ The elephant penis is muscular type, similar to that of horses and humans.
- ➤ It is S-shaped when fully erect and has a Y-shaped orifice.
- ➤ Musth, a rapid increase in the androgen level and secretion from temporal glands, characterized by aggression and excitement, is seen in male Asian elephants. Musth can last up to 3 months, and elephant can be calmed using antiandrogens like flutamide.
- ➤ Manual semen collection and artificial insemination techniques have been standardized for Asian elephants in an effort to increase the population.

Female
- ➤ Uterine horns are bilateral, similar to the cow, with ovaries placed behind the kidneys.
- ➤ The genital canal can be 68-88 cm long.
- ➤ The vulva is 40 cm long and positioned between the inguinal regions, ventrally, unlike perineal position seen in other mammals.
- ➤ The clitoris is as long as vulva.
- ➤ Elephants have two mammary glands located pectorally between the forelimbs.
- ➤ The placenta of the elephant is zonary.
- ➤ The typical gestation period of the elephant is 17-22 months, with male calf averaging 21-24 months and female calf averaging 17-23 months.
- ➤ The normal estrous cycle of the Asian elephant is between 14 and 18 weeks, that is 3 cycles in a year, with luteal phase lasting 10-14 weeks and follicular phase lasting 3-6 weeks.
- ➤ Follicular phase is characterized by 2 surges of luteinizing hormone occurring 3 weeks apart, with the first surge being anovulatory (anLH), and ovulation occurring around 24 hours after the second LH (ovLH) surge.
- ➤ The importance of double LH surge is still not understood.

- The fertile period starts 2 days before ovulation and lasts up to a short time after ovulation.
- Signs of pregnancy are not marked, and fetal movements can be appreciated externally by 12th month.
- Process of birth resembles that seen in domestic herbivores.
- Immediately after birth, mother throws sand on offspring to clear placental debris.
- Newborn urinates, defecates, stands, walks and suckles within one hour unassisted by the mother.
- The average birth weight of calves is 80-100 kg.
- Twinning is also commonly seen.

Eye

- Elephants do not have a lacrimal apparatus.
- Hardarian glands, which maintain the moisture on the eye, can be observed close to the third eyelid. The third eyelid is well developed and is strong enough to protect the globe of the eye.
- The pupil and iris are circular shaped, with iris colored greenish-brown and blue.
- Because of large ears, trunk and limited mobility of the eyes, elephants have poor vision.

Ear

- The ear of the elephant is thick at the base and thin at the tips, and are second most important sense organ.
- The elephant can hear at 12,000 Hertz in the upper limit, compared to bats (80,000 Hertz), dogs (40,000 Hertz) and humans (20,000 Hertz). These differences make elephant communications inaudible to human ears.

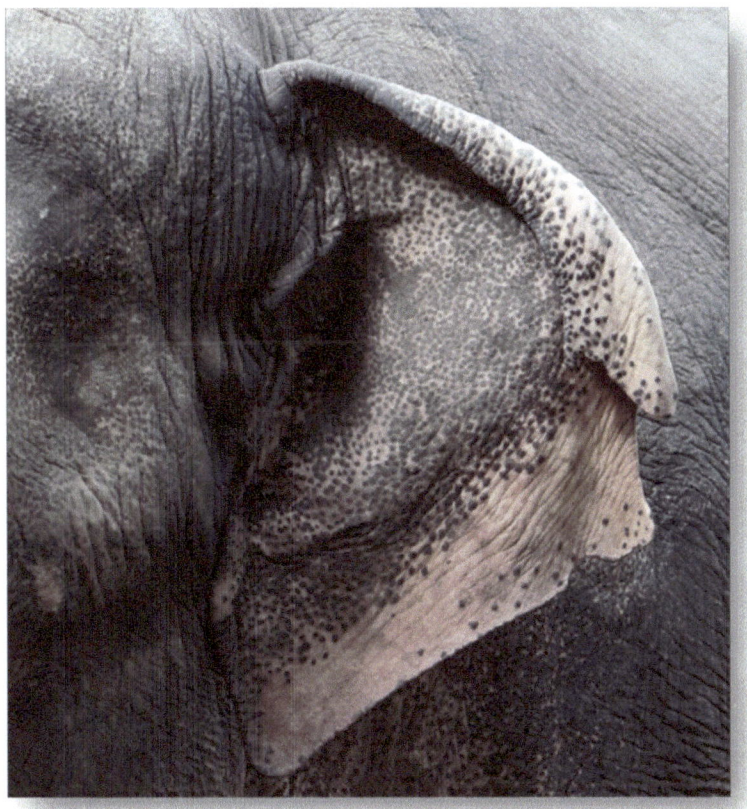

Figure 11: Inward curling of ear with age in an Asian elephant.
Image by Tuxyso, used under creative commons attribution.
http://upload.wikimedia.org/wikipedia/commons/thumb/8/89/Elephas-maximus-Ear.jpg/427px-
Elephas-maximus-Ear.jpg

> ➤ They can communicate with other elephants at a great distance using these ultrasonic wavelengths.
> ➤ Apart from acoustic functions, the ears help with balance, thermoregulation and information transfer.
> ➤ Temperature dependent vasoconstriction in auricular blood vessels plays a major role in elephant thermoregulation.
> ➤ Elephant ear pinna curls 1 inch every 30 years, which can be used to approximate its age.

Chapter 3

MANAGEMENT OF CAPTIVE ASIAN ELEPHANTS

Management strategies for elephants should be formulated considering its wild nature, anatomical and physiological features and cost factors. Successful captive management of elephant starts when a calf is born, which has to be nursed properly and handed over to an affectionate mahout during weaning, who can psychologically replace its mother and impart all trainings as well as take care of its health and basic needs throughout its life.

Housing Aspects

All the basic principles like sufficient space, hygiene, aeration, safety, easy management, etc. should be considered during the housing of elephants. The house should be cleaned frequently of leftover food, urine, feces and other waste materials. Minimum space requirements vary with age as below:

Category	Floor space requirement (In meters)
Adult elephant	9X5
Cow elephant with calf	9X5
Weaned calf	5X2.5
Sub-adult elephant	7X3.5

Compiled from K.S. Subramania. Veterinary management of captive Asian elephants. Published by Tamil Nadu Veterinary and Animal Sciences University. 2010.

Feeding Aspects

Food is the most important management aspect for elephants as they have large requirement and poor digestibility.

Improper feeding may lead to unpredictable destructive behavioral episodes in addition to loss of health.

Based on the nature of elephant rearing, food can be completely natural, completely cultivated or a mix of the two. Elephants eat more than 200 varieties of plants in natural habitat, which ensures balanced nutrition. Natural food can be cheaper, more nutritious and free from chemical contaminants. However, with time, the number of captive or semi-captive elephants is increasing and it is not always possible to provide natural food completely. Feeding cultivated food reduces the diversity of dietary components and exposes elephants to chemicals in addition to enhanced cost. Further, the quantity of food may also be reduced. Mahouts should be taught about the importance of a balanced diet and should be given freedom to feed natural plants or grasses whenever possible. All the feed items should be subjected to quality checks routinely.

In addition to the anatomical and physiological features, following behavioral aspects has to be considered while formulating a feeding plan for captive elephants

- ➢ The elephant is a simple stomached herbivore, with digestive system resembling that of the horse.
- ➢ The stomach has a capacity of holding 200 to 300 kg. of food.
- ➢ The flexures in the large intestine are the site of constipation and colic.
- ➢ Elephants require roughage at the rate of about 5 % of its body weight and 200-250 liters of drinking water every day.
- ➢ In natural habitats, elephants spend about 20 hours in a day on feeding, as the digestive system is less efficient and requirement is high.
- ➢ Elephants eat a large variety of plant materials in a rhythmic pattern.
- ➢ Elephants also prefer to eat soil rich in minerals periodically.
- ➢ Trunk, mouth and lower lips are used for prehensile act, whereas only molars are used to grind the feed.

➢ Tusk and forelegs are used to collect and position the feed for intake.

➢ A specialized structure of the teeth allows breakage of even toughest plant materials.

➢ Undigested food and residues are expelled after 24 hours, which can continue up to 50 hrs after ingestion.

➢ The food is mixed with large amounts of saliva and esophageal secretions to digest and lubricate.

➢ Up to 70% of the feed is held in cecum for fermentation by anaerobic microbes and fungi. The feed is broken into volatile fatty acids with approximate ratio of 75:12:10 (acetate: propionate: butyrate).

➢ The digestibility of Asian elephants for various feed ingredients is: 45% to 51% for dry matter, 18% for crude fiber and crude protein. Free ranging animals have higher digestibility compared to captive elephants.

➢ Care must be taken to properly cook the concentrates.

➢ Concentrates should be fed in two equal parts during the morning and evening.

➢ Feed should be given after bath and before taking elephants to work.

➢ Elephants like to take time to eat.

➢ Providing water immediately after feeding and other such improper practices can lead to serious health problems.

➢ Some special considerations about feeding elephants
  o Captive elephants fed on palm leaves alone should be supplemented with 30-60 g of phosphorus every day.
  o Calcium should be supplemented at the rate of 8-9 g/day for tuskers and 60 g/day for lactating mothers.
  o Elephants have a high affinity to sodium rich water and soil.
  o Vitamin E and other vitamin deficiency are common in captive elephants, which can be avoided by supplementing.

➤ Calves can be weaned at the completion of 3 years. However, weaning can be done after 2 years if excellent food and care was provided. Males can be separated earlier than females due to early development of temperament suitable for smooth weaning.

➤ Sometimes orphan calves need to be hand reared, which is a very difficult task, and requires formulation of special food considering the following points:

   o Elephant produce milk similar to humans, which is difficult to obtain.

   o Elephant calves, especially younger than one month, cannot tolerate cow's milk easily as fat droplets are comparatively larger.

   o Characteristics of elephant milk are as below

Particulars	Normal value
Specific gravity	1.02 to 1.03
Solids (%)	16.4 to 28.5
Ash (%)	0.6 to 0.8
Fat (%)	6 to 19
Protein (%)	4.4 to 5.4
Casein (%)	1.4 to 2.5
Lactose (%)	3.4 to 5.4
Calcium (mg%)	84 to 180
Chloride (mg%)	42 to 64
Phosphate (mg%)	186 to 310
Vitamin C (mg%)	0.25 to 4.0
pH	8 to 9

Compiled from Healthcare Management of Captive Asian Elephants, Eds. Ajitkumar and others, Faculty of Veterinary and Animal Sciences, Kerala Agricultural University, Kerala 2009.

   o If calves show diarrhea, milk should be replaced as it indicates intolerance.

   o Hygiene principles should be followed as immunity will be poor in calves.

o A simple rice based formulation commonly used in India is made by whole milk powder (500 g), cooked brown rice (500 g), sucrose (200 g), water (8.5 l), and bone meal at the rate of 825 mg/100g of food. Vitamin and mineral concentrate should also be included. Elephant milk is rich in Capric acid, which can be supplemented by including coconut oil or coconut water.

Training

➢ As soon as the animal is received for captive management, age dependent training schedule has to be initiated to help the animal accommodate in captive management lifestyle.
➢ During the last days in kraal, elephant has to be trained for obedience, direction of movement, firm placement of feet on the ground.
➢ After taking out of the kraal, with the association of the Koonkie elephants, other routine skills like bathing, walking and standing in the presence of people, fodder carrying, timber hauling etc has to be imparted over a period of 1 to 2 years.
➢ Timber hauling and standing in processions should be taught to elephants older than 5 years with a height of more than 1.8 m.

Table 1: A general feeding outline followed for forest camp elephants.

Ingredient	Up to 1 year			1 to 4 years		4 to 20 years			More than 20 years			
									Maintenance period		Working period	
	<3 months	3 to 6 months	6 to 12 months	1 to 2 years	2 to 4 years	4 to 7 years	7 to 12 years	12 to 20 years	Male	Female	Male	Female
Milk (liters)	10			Nil								
Ragi (Kg)	2 (baby formulation)	Nil	4	3	3	4	6	6	2	2	7	7
Horse Gram (Kg)	Nil	Nil	1	1	2	2	3	4	2	1	5	4
Wheat/Rice (Kg)		1	1		2	2	3	3	2	1	3	3
Common Salt (gm)	10	15	20	50	50	100	100	100	100	100	100	100
Mineral mixture (gm)	20	25	25	50	75	100	100	100	100	100	100	100
Jaggery (gm)	500	250	250	200	100	100	150	200	50	50	50	50
Green Fodder (Coconut	Nil	5	10	50	100	150	200	250	250	250	250	250

leaves/palm leaves, kg)						
Glucose (gm)	500	250		Nil		
Complan (gm, divided into 2 servings)	100			Nil		
Coconut milk	2 medium sized coconuts			Nil		
Ashtachoornam (gm, 4 days in a week)	50					
Drinking water	Ad libitum					

Compiled from Healthcare Management of Captive Asian Elephants, Eds. Ajitkumar and others, Faculty of Veterinary and Animal Sciences, Kerala Agricultural University, Kerala 2009.

Special considerations about working elephants

➢ Age of the elephant and the nature of work should be considered before work assignments.
➢ Animals should be worked preferably during cool hours.
➢ Elephants should not be loaded more than following specifications (inclusive of gears, mahout or trainer) according to their height:

Load carrying		Timber hauling	
<1.5 m	Not used	<2.1 m	Not used
1.5 to 1.8 m	≤150 kg	2.1 to 2.25 m	Dragging of timber <750 kg
1.8 to 2.25 m	≤200 kg	>2.25 m	Dragging of timber ≤1000 kg
2.25 to 2.55 m	≤300 kg		
>2.55 m	≤400 kg		

Compiled from K.S. Subramania. Veterinary management of captive Asian elephants. Published by Tamil Nadu Veterinary and Animal Sciences University. 2010.

Precautions during transport of elephants

➢ Food and water schedule should be maintained by carrying in sufficient quantity and planning refills en-route.
➢ One truck with length more than 12 feet can be used to carry a maximum of two weaned calves (of less than 1.5 m height), or one cow elephant with a un-weaned calf, or one sub-adult/adult (of height more than 1.5 m).
➢ A rest of 12 hours should be given every 12 hours.
➢ Pregnant, sick and elephants in musth should not be transported.
➢ In case of long distance transport, trains should be preferred.

- ➢ Each wagon should be accompanied by at least two mahouts.
- ➢ Sedatives can be used to prevent excitement.
- ➢ On foot, elephants should not be walked continuously for more than 3 hours.
- ➢ On foot, elephants should not be transported more than 30 km.
- ➢ Journeys longer than 50 km should be conducted by truck or rails.

Musth and its management

- ➢ Healthy male Asian elephants aged more than 18 years undergo a natural hormonal change, usually same time every year, a phenomenon called musth.
- ➢ Elephants in musth, with some exceptions, become stubborn, dangerous and aggressive for a period of 1 to 4 months. Aggression can be either specific towards humans or elephants or non-specific towards anything, including mahout.
- ➢ Younger elephants aged less than 15 years show a mild form of musth called "moda musth", "grass musth" or "honey musth" which is characterized by honey colored temporal gland secretion. Four to five years after this, elephants exhibit true musth.

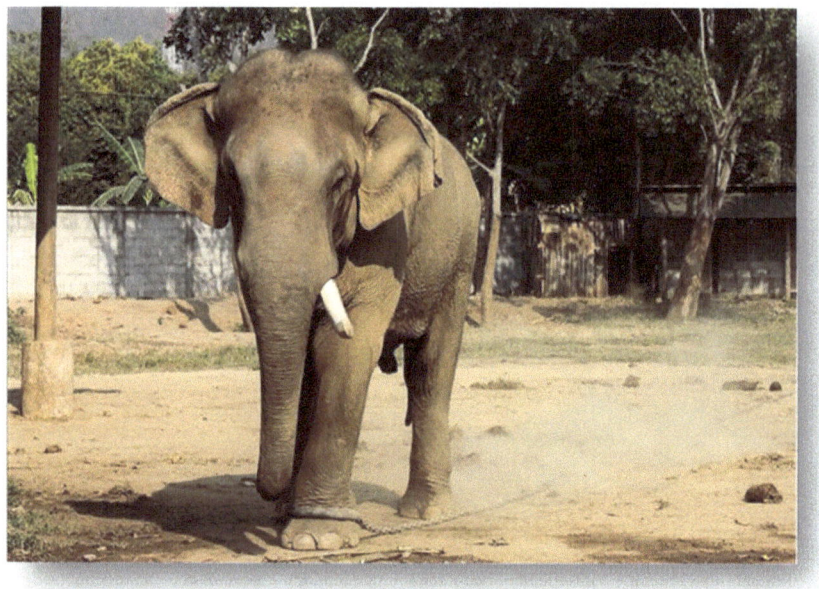

Figure 1: A Thai elephant in musth. Image by OXOX, used under creative commons attribution.
http://upload.wikimedia.org/wikipedia/commons/b/b9/Thai_bull_elephant_in_musth.jpg

> Musth has 3 phases

1. *Coming into musth (1 to 5 days):* characterized by thickening of neck, fattening, swelling of and secretion of temporal glands, stubbornness and disobedience, heightened alertness, staring at anything for long periods, frequent erections, dribbling of urine, and loss of appetite.
2. *Full musth (1 to 5 months):* characterized by increased swelling of the temporal glands with the secretion of a tarry colored smelly fluid, continuous erection with secretion of accessory sex glands, increased aggression, failure to recognize even mahout.
3. *End of musth (2 weeks to 2 months):* characterized by reduction of temporal secretion with shrinkage of the

glands, elephant slowly returns to normal state as before.

➢ Sometimes healthy and fatty female elephants also come into "grass musth", under the influence of stressful situation like the birth of a calf.

➢ *Special considerations during management of elephants in musth:* At the initiation of the earliest symptoms of musth, following preparations should be undertaken to successfully manage the elephant in musth.

  o A quiet, isolated, cool, even, smooth, clean, strong and shaded tethering site has to be identified. If possible, this site should be adjacent to flowing clean water, which elephant can drink and use for bathing.

  o Keep other elephants as well as people not associated with this elephant away from the musth elephant.

  o Tethering site should be slightly sloped to facilitate drainage of urine and rain water. Alternatively, an area containing clean soil, which can absorb the urine and is easy to clean can be used.

  o All the materials used for musth elephant should be strong enough to withstand elephant's aggression and should be thoroughly inspected before use.

  o To reduce the intensity and duration of musth, the energy level of the diet can be reduced without altering other nutrients. Instead of rice, ragi and calorie rich items, succulent and fiber rich foods like banana tree stalks, dried grass etc. can be given. This will reduce the amount of energy in the food without reducing the total quantity consumed.

  o In case of uncontrollable aggression, antiandrogens like flutamide can be given to negate the behavioral effects.

Approximation of age

> ➢ Age of the elephants can be roughly estimated based on physical features and dentition.
> ➢ The number of laminae on each molar can be used to identify the age of the elephant

Molar set	Laminaes	Appearance/grinding age	Replacement/worn out age
1	4	4 months	2-2.5 yrs
2	8	6 months	6 yrs
3	12	3 years	9 yrs
4	12 (broad)	6 years	25 yrs
5	16	20 years	50-60 yrs
6	24	40 years	Lifelong

(Modified and compiled from Healthcare Management of Captive Asian Elephants, Eds. Ajitkumar and others, Faculty of Veterinary and Animal Sciences, Kerala Agricultural University, Kerala 2009)

Physical characteristics useful in approximation of age in Asian elephants			
Feature	Less than 12 years	13 to 45 years	Over 46 years
Dung	Fine textured		Coarse with undigested food materials
Ears	No curls at top or no cuts at bottom.	Forward curls on top and some tears at bottom.	Deep forward curls on top with numerous cuts on the lower side.
Feet and nails	Foot and ankle circumference similar. Smooth toenails.	Foot circumference larger than ankle. Smooth toenails. Foot-pad without	Circumference of foot much larger than ankle. Toenails chalky, rough and spread

		cracks.	apart.
Head	Temples are smooth. Skin fits tightly.	Temples are slightly depressed. Skin fits tightly.	Temples are deeply concave.
Muscles	Strong and bundled.		Flabby and week
Skin	Thick, taut, smooth, supple and evenly pigmented.	Thick, not very wrinkled and supple to touch.	Wrinkled, droopy rough and dry.
Tail	Orderly tail hairs. Not kinked or knotty.		Knotty with few tail hairs

Compiled from Preecha Phuangkum, Richard C. Lair and Taweepoke Angkawanith. Elephant care manual for mahouts and camp managers. Forest industry organization, Ministry of natural resources and environment, Food and agriculture organization of the united nations, Regional office for Asia and the pacific Bangkok, 2005.

Approximation of weight

➤ Estimation of weight is required for planning routine management practices and calculation of dosage of medicine. Numerous formulae are available for estimation of the weight of Indian elephants, however the equations by Kurt (2002) are recent and good for sex specific weight estimation:
  - BW = HT.CG2/10000 up to 6 years of age
  - BW = 0.93 X HT.CG2/10000 for <6 year males
  - BW = 0.98 X HT.CG2/10000 for >6 year female
  - Where BW is in kg, HT and CG are in centimeters.

➤ The following measurements are used to estimate the weight
  - Height at shoulders (HT): A tape is fixed to a straight rod and the rod is placed parallel to the ground on the shoulder of the elephant. The minimum distance

between the rod and the ground is called height at shoulders.

- o Chest girth (CG): Circumference of chest measured by encircling the tape tightly around the body, just behind the elbows.
- o Neck girth (NG): Circumference of neck measured by encircling the tape tightly at the base of the neck, in front of the shoulders.
- o Body length (L1): The head to tail distance, i.e., the distance between the base of the forehead (midpoint of the supraoccipital crest) along the curvature of the back to the base of the tail.
- o Body length (L2): Point of buttock (tuber ischii) to point of shoulder (greater tuberosity of the humerus) length.
- o Forefoot circumference (FFC): Circumference at the level of the sole including the nail.

Veterinary care

Timely vaccination, de-worming and treatment of ailments should be undertaken.

Retirement of elephants

Elephants above the age of 65 years are retired from work, however, if they are healthy, they can be put into light work.

Chapter 4

HEALTHCARE OF ASIAN ELEPHANT

The health of the elephants can be appreciated by body condition and behavior. Similar to domestic animals, assessment of specific health conditions should be based on laboratory tests.

General features of a healthy Asian elephant

- A healthy elephant, except the baby, sleeps only after midnight
- Aware of and alert to the surroundings
- Bright and moist eyes with no abnormal discharge
- Ear and tail movements most of the times
- Mucosa of the oral cavity, tongue, tip of the trunk, anus and vulva will be bright pink
- Normal appetite and digestion
- Smooth and supple skin with normal hydration
- Sweating on the coronet line above the toenail
- Yellow colored urination and greenish defecation without hard or liquid consistency

General features of a sick Asian elephant

- Inappetite or anorexia
- Lethargy, frequent yawning, sleepy and slow movements of trunk and tail
- Non sweating coronet
- Slow and lethargic ear movements
- Tries to sleep daytime or in standing position
- Weight loss, especially in young elephant

- Dull skin, blotches on the body
- Reduced urination
- Abnormal colored urine and feces
- Hard dung coated with mucus.

General Physical Examination of Asian elephant

Visual inspection

Elephants should be observed daily in the morning just after waking up from sleep from a distance when they are involved in their routine activities. Its environment should also be observed with special emphasis on sleeping place, food, water, urine, feces, etc. Following aspects can be covered by these observations:
- Feeding and drinking
- Walking and gait
- Sleep and alertness
- Response to environmental stimuli
- Urination and defecation
- Ear, tail, trunk and other body part movements
- Noise

Physical examination

Visually observed features can be confirmed by physical observation, which has to be done in the presence of its mahout. The veterinarian should maintain a safe distance from the elephants during all examinations
- *Palpation*: Palpation can be done to inspect for abnormal mass, growth, size, injury, pain etc.
- *Percussion*: Can be done to test the repercussions of internal organs.
- *Auscultation*: Can be done with a stethoscope, by maintaining quietness during examination. Fatty elephants may be difficult examine.
- *Smelling*: Foul or bad smells can be detected by close observation.

➤ *Pulse rate*: Arteries on the back of the ear can be used to read the pulse rate. Ranges from 28/min in standing to 35/min during recumbency.

➤ *Respiratory rate:* Respiration is difficult to read from nostrils, instead abdominal movements can be counted to find the rate of respiration. Ranges from 10/min in standing to 5/min on recumbency.

➤ *Temperature*: Rectal temperature can be taken by wearing gloves and inserting thermometer with the assistance of mahout when the animal is recumbent. The thermometer has to be held for 1-2 minutes to obtain a stable reading. In case of non-cooperative elephants freshly expelled dung can be used to read the temperature, by inserting the tip deep into the boli for 1-2 minutes. Reading taken from feces should be increased by 1° C to obtain body temperature.

➤ Urine will be turbid and alkaline with a volume exceeding 50 liters in a day.

Clinical Examination

Hematology

Hematological examination is conducted for diagnosis of nutritional, metabolic and infectious diseases.

➤ Some special features of elephant blood are
  o Elephants have largest erythrocytes, and in effect highest hemoglobin content, among terrestrial animals.
  o Hematology should also consider age, sex and environmental conditions.
  o Panic increases the neutrophil and lymphocyte count.
  o Young ones have more leukocytes than adults.
  o Compared to other animals, elephants have a higher platelet count, and in effect, lower clotting times (about 5.5 Sec).

Blood Chemistry

For evaluating function of visceral organs, like liver, kidneys, muscle, etc. and nutritional status biochemical parameters can be evaluated.

Urinalysis

Can be performed as a noninvasive method for understanding renal health. Should be performed before giving medicines.

Fecal Examination

Routine and need based fecal examination should be performed to monitor parasitic infections.

Table 1: Certain features of blood of Indian Elephants

Constituents	Baby elephant	Tuskers	Adult non-lactating non-pregnant females
Specific gravity			
Whole blood	1.05	1.054	1.054
Plasma	1.02	1.027	1.028
Relative viscosity	6.37	6.1	6.36
Absolute viscosity	5.7	5.54	5.68
Whole blood coagulation time	5.39	6.71	5.3
Serum Icterus index	2.29	2.24	2.25

Compiled from K.S. Subramania. Veterinary management of captive Asian elephants. Published by Tamil Nadu Veterinary and Animal Sciences University. 2010.

Radiography and Ultrasonography

- ➢ Radiography can be conducted to detect fracture of tusk and legs (babies) under good restrain.
- ➢ Care should be taken to protect genitalia and thyroid organs.

> ➤ Ultrasonography can be conducted for assessment of the reproductive system, gastrointestinal system and ocular functioning.

Table 2: Normal hematological values of India elephants

Constituent	Baby elephant	Tuskers	Adult		
			Non- lactating non- pregnant females	Pregnant	Lactating
RBC (million/cu.m	2.42	2.47	2.4	1.84	2.65
Hemoglobin (g%)	11.12	10.24	10.72	9.98	11.1
VPRC (%)	34.7	34.8	34.8	29.8	33.5
MCV (fl)	144.8	142	146.9	168.6	126.5
MCH (pg)	46.67	46.93	44.49	56.93	41.9
MCHC (g%)	32.13	29.69	31.06	33.77	33.14
ESR (mm/hr)	61.3	63.4	61.3	67.4	64.5
WBC/μl	11900	8780	9810	12400	8900
Neutrophils	32.1	34.2	32.3	44.1	35
Eosinophils	3.8	6.2	6.6	1.9	4
Basophils (%)	0.6	0.7	0.9	0.5	1
Lymphocytes	59	52.8	56.2	50.6	54
Monocytes	4.5	6.07	3.9	2.9	6

Compiled from Healthcare Management of Captive Asian Elephants, Eds. Ajitkumar and others, Faculty of Veterinary and Animal Sciences, Kerala Agricultural University, Kerala 2009.

Table 3: Blood biochemical measurements of Indian elephants

| Constituent | Baby elephant | Tuskers | Adult | | |
			Non-lactating non-pregnant females	Pregnant	Lactating
Total cholesterol (mg%)	116.68	111.38	93.66	130.83	115.13
Inorganic phosphate (mg%)	5.54	4.47	4.07	4.4	4.27
Glucose (mg%)	67.47	59.54	52.86	62.5	64
Chloride (mg%)	473.6	488	496.9	510	433
Sodium (mmol/l)	125.36	118.2	126.99	—	—
Potassium	4.97	4.77	4.85	—	—
Calcium (mg%)	12.2	11.8	12.5	11.1	11.1
Magnesium	2.41	2.06	2.33	2.68	2.49
Copper (μmol/l)	23.84	28.74	33.69	—	—
Iron (μmol/l)	34.78	44.48	43.26	—	—
Zinc (μmol/l)	31.13	33.73	42.61	—	—
Iron: Copper ratio	1.5	1.14	1.33	—	—

Compiled from K.S. Subramania. Veterinary management of captive Asian elephants. Published by Tamil Nadu Veterinary and Animal Sciences University. 2010.

Table 4: Normal plasma protein characteristics of Indian elephants

Constituent	Baby elephant	Tuskers	Adult non-pregnant, non-	Pregnant	Lactating
Total protein	8.25	8.49	9.25	7.99	9.28
Albumin	2.2	2.36	2.1	2.08	2.06
Globulin	5.41	5.56	6.5	5.32	6.68
A/G ratio	0.45	0.46	0.34	0.42	0.33
Fibrinogen (g%)	0.64	0.57	0.65	0.58	0.54

Compiled from Healthcare Management of Captive Asian Elephants, Eds. Ajitkumar and others, Faculty of Veterinary and Animal Sciences, Kerala Agricultural University, Kerala 2009.

Table 5: Serum enzyme activity in Indian elephants

Constituent	Baby elephant	Tuskers	Adult non pregnant, non-lactating
AST (SGOT) (U/L)	10.2	15.7	18.5
ALT (SGPT) (U/L)	5.6	4.8	5
LDH (U/L)	366.7	468.8	398.8
CK (U/L)	30.3	51.2	43.8
AKP (Bodansky	—	—	1.25
ACP (Bodansky	—	—	0.35
Amylase (Somogyi	—	—	381.09

Compiled from Healthcare Management of Captive Asian Elephants, Eds. Ajitkumar and others, Faculty of Veterinary and Animal Sciences, Kerala Agricultural University, Kerala 2009.

Points to consider when dealing with an elephant

➢ Always take extra care while dealing with elephants as they are massive and unpredictable.

➢ Learn the behavioral characteristics and complete history about the elephant before handling it.

➢ Do not work with unrestrained elephants, if not at least make sure that mahout has complete control over the elephant.

➢ Call the name of the elephant or make soft sounds throughout the handling duration.

➢ Examine the elephant only in the presence of the mahout.

➢ Stay in the safe zone around the elephant and away from the trunk as much as possible.

➢ Elephants can use tail to beat a person, so it has to be secured while working around the hindquarters.

➢ Limbs should be secured separately during examination.

➢ Do not stand in between the limbs when an elephant is recumbent.

➢ Do not show medical instruments to elephants as they can recall previous experiences and react.

➢ Analgesia or sedatives should be used for conducting painful procedures.

Points to be considered while darting a rogue elephant

➢ Make sure whether the elephant is in musth.
➢ Keep safe distance all the times.
➢ Take help of and suggestions from experienced mahouts and elephant owners.
➢ Complete the legal paperwork before beginning the operation.
➢ Estimate the body weight of the animal from a distance and prepare a dart and antidote based on it and keep it ready for use.
➢ In some situations, the elephant may be under partial or total restraint and if the animal is trying to break the chain, take measures to reinforce it.
➢ Inform the police for control of the mob and maintain calm.
➢ While approaching the animal for darting, hide the syringe projector from the animal and select a convenient and safe place to stand with the syringe projector for darting.
➢ Darting should be avoided during evening and night times.
➢ Darting should not be done in uneven terrains and near water bodies.
➢ If the mahout or the public is sitting on the back of the elephant, extreme care should be taken to avoid darting them.
➢ Elephants run for a distance in forward direction after hit by a dart, this must be considered when planning the operation.
➢ As it is difficult to assure whether the medicine is delivered after successful darting, a time of twenty minutes has to be given to observe and confirm the delivery.
➢ The classical signs of sedation are complete relaxation of the penis, standing fixed at a place, lack of movements of the ears and trunk, sleepy appearance, snoring etc.

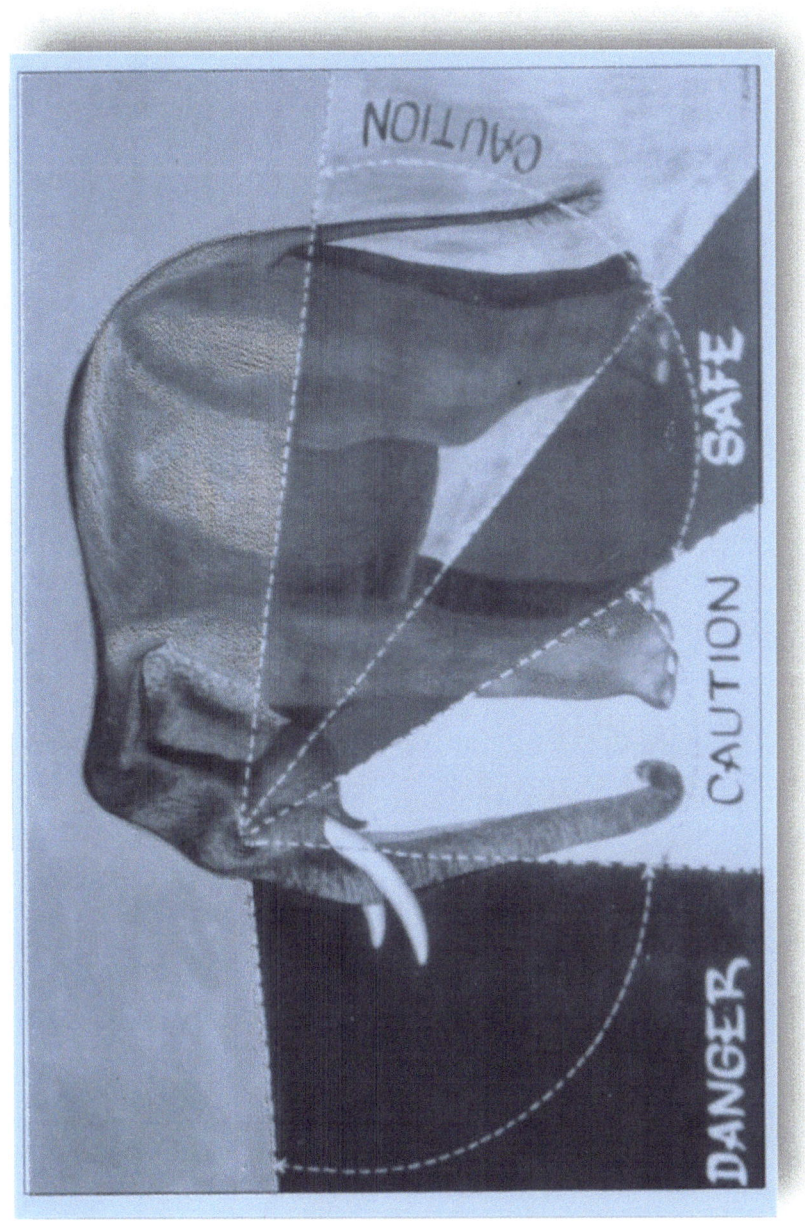

Figure 1: Safety around elephants. (Modified and adapted from Healthcare Management of Captive Asian Elephants, Eds. Ajitkumar and others, Faculty of Veterinary and Animal Sciences, Kerala Agricultural University, Kerala 2009)

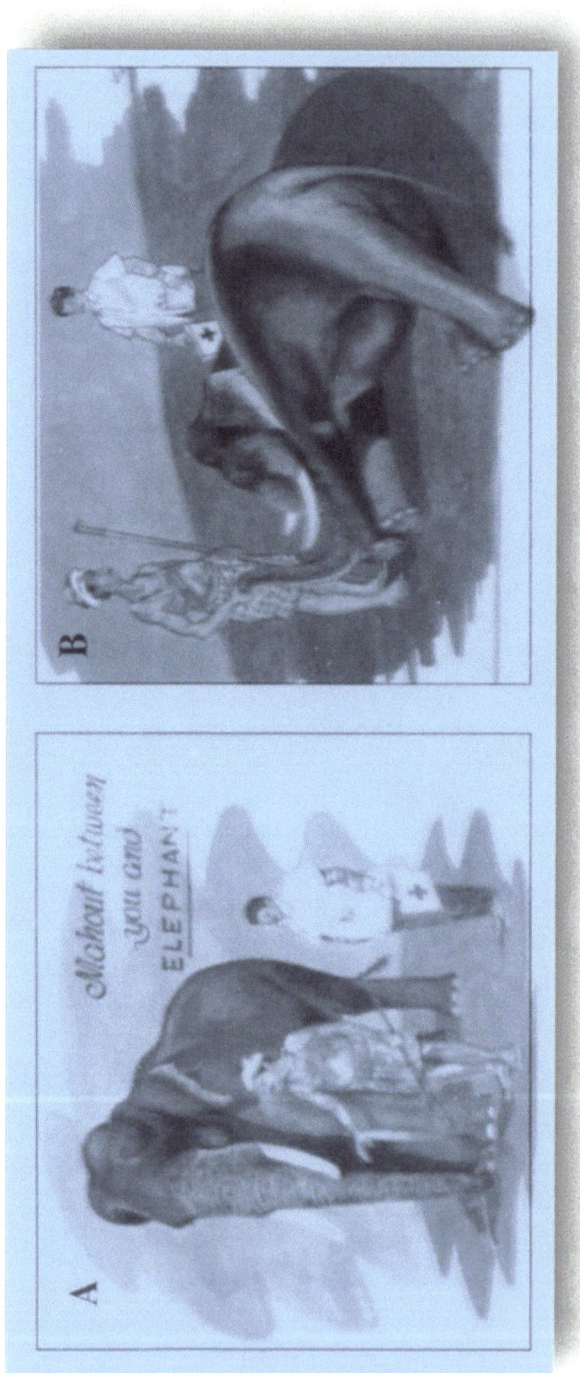

Figure 2: Safe position for veterinary examinations. Note that mahout should accompany during examination in standing (A) as well as sitting (B) position. (Modified and adapted from Healthcare Management of Captive Asian Elephants, Eds. Ajitkumar and others, Faculty of Veterinary and Animal Sciences, Kerala Agricultural University, Kerala 2009)

> ➤ When an elephant is overdosed and signs like, trying to lay down with a relaxed penis, feeling very sleepy, are observed the antidote should be administered immediately.
> ➤ Translocate the sedated animal to a shade and tether to a strong tree.
> ➤ If the elephant comes out of sedation, second dose may be darted accordingly.

Administration of medicines in elephants

All administrations have to be done after securing the elephant and only in the presence of the mahout who can control the elephant during the procedure.

Intramuscular injection
> ➤ Intramuscular injection can be administered in the triangular region of the neck, between shoulder and elbow region and buttock region.
> ➤ A needle of 18-16 G and minimum length of 1.5 inches should be used.
> ➤ Perfect asepsis should be maintained during the injection as elephants easily develop an abscess at injecting sites.
> ➤ The needle can be inserted at right angles to the skin.
> ➤ At a single site, a maximum of 50 ml of clear liquid or 20 ml of suspension or oil adjuvant based formulation can be administered.
> ➤ Administration should be preferred in a recumbent position with limbs placed stretched and straight.
> ➤ Gluteal region should be the first priority for injection.

Subcutaneous injection
> ➤ It is uncommon to use the subcutaneous route as elephants are prone to abscess formation.

> However, certain drugs like antricide and ivermectin has to be given by this route.
> Loose skin folds on the sides of the base of the tail are preferred for this route.
> Care should be taken to avoid intradermal delivery.

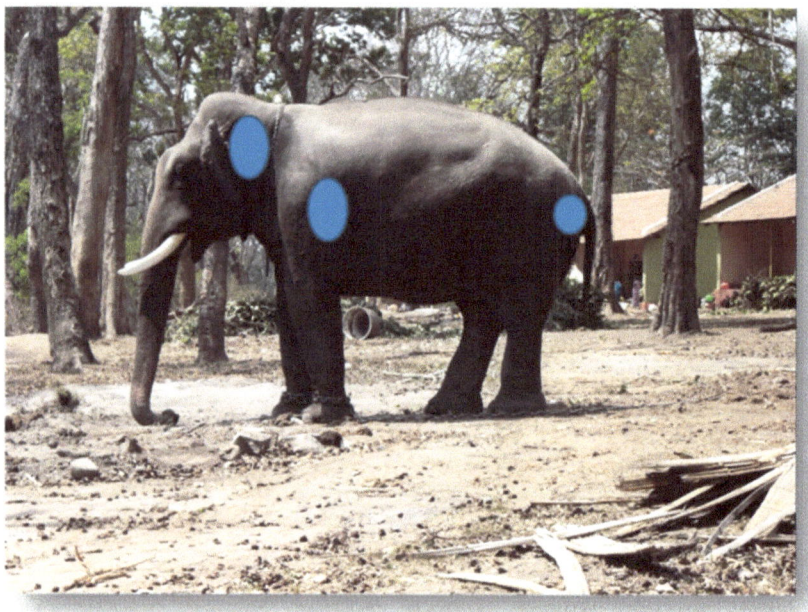

Figure 3: Sites of intramuscular administration in elephants.
Picture by Madhukar Dama.

Intravenous injection
> Soft veins on the hind side of the ear pinnae are preferred for intravenous injections and fluid therapy.
> The vein can be blocked with fingers to raise the thickness and see it clearly.
> The animal should be restrained on lateral recumbency for this procedure. However, if possible, it can be done in standing position also.
> The ear pinna should be washed with plenty of water, dried thoroughly and sterilized with 60% tincture iodine or ethyl alcohol before puncture.

➢ The ear should be folded anteriorly and secured tightly at the tip.

➢ Arteries should be identified and avoided.

➢ Stainless steel needle of 14-16 G or IV canula of the same size can be used.

➢ Avoid subcutaneous delivery of the formulation.

➢ Glycerine-magsulph paste can be applied after administration to reduce the inflammation.

➢ In colder climates, warm water washing can help raise the veins.

➢ Alternatively, saphenous vein on the inner side of the hind limb can also be used for intravenous administration.

Oral medication

➢ Baby elephants can be forcefully administered medicine by oral route.

➢ Oral administration in adults is a difficult task as elephants are very sensitive to smell and taste.

➢ During training periods, elephants can be frequently given tasty boli without medication to simulate oral medication, so that it will cooperate when a bad tasting boli need to be given.

➢ Later, this same boli can be given with the medication.

➢ Commonly used boli for administration of oral medicine for Indian elephants are cooked plain rice balls, cooked rice-jaggery balls, plain jiggery, pineapple, apple, banana, bread loaves, etc.

➢ Docile elephants can allow confirmation of ingestion of boli, whereas it should not be attempted in aggressive elephants.

➢ The tablet should be hidden in the center of the boli for administration, to conceal its taste.

➢ For liquids, silicon tube or syringe can be used.

Subconjunctival injection

➢ It is used in conditions like corneal opacity

➢ Elephants have a prominent third eyelid, which prevents access to subconjunctiva through the palpebral fissure.

➢ Subconjunctival injection can be given by inserting needle from the outer side of the upper eyelid parallel to the palpebral fissure.

Common diseases encountered in Indian elephants

Bacterial Diseases

➢ *Tuberculosis*: Tuberculosis is a chronic disease caused by *Mycobacterium tuberculosis*, which usually enters the body trough trunk, windpipe and lungs. It is believed that the elephants are more susceptible to human type of *M. tuberculosis*. Clinical symptoms develop over a long time, maybe two years after entry of the organism. The elephants suffering from tuberculosis show the symptoms such as anorexia, progressive weakness, and foul smelling thick yellowish discharge from trunk, lethargy and rapid exhaustion. Trunk wash can be collected for confirming the diagnosis. Intramuscular administration of Streptomycin at a dose of 100 gm on alternate days for a period of four weeks is useful. Oral administration of 30 capsules (each containing Rifamycin 450 mg and isoniazid 300 mg) twice daily for a period of 6-12 months is found to be effective in controlling symptoms in chronic cases. Suspected elephants should be separated immediately from other elephants. Annual inspection of health, including chest X rays of all mahouts, caretakers and other persons involved is necessary as TB is a zoonotically important.

➢ *Tetanus*: Tetanus is usually found in elephants that have suffered deep wounds, usually in the foot and particularly through the foot pad after being pierced by metal objects such as an old, rusty nail. This condition is caused by infection with *Clostridium tetani* and is characterized by partial or complete locked jaw, inability to drink water, stiffness of limbs, paroxysms and jerky movements of the muscles and high mortality rate. The tail has a supple, snakelike appearance. Periodic spasms can also be observed. Animals die because of locked jay which disables feeding and drinking. Though the disease is believed to be incurable, a solitary case of tetanus was treated successfully by administering Diazepam, tetanus serum (2.5 lakh units), Crystalline Penicillin (450 lank units) and a combination of electrolytes and dextrose (25 liters). This treatment needs to be repeated on subsequent day also.

➤ *Anthrax*: This disease is caused by *Bacillus anthracis* and its incidence is comparatively less in domesticated elephants. The characteristic features of this disease are the sudden onset, grave general disturbance, high body temperature, hemorrhage from the trunk, some time blood stained dung and urine, swelling of the throat behind the ears, etc. The affected elephant should be isolated as quickly as possible and all other elephants should be moved as far away as possible. Highly nutritious and tempting food such as ripe bananas, sugarcane, and green grass should be offered. Penicillin is the drug of choice in this case. If it is clear that the animal is going to die, but it can still walk, one should move it to a site where disposal is more convenient and to prevent spread of infection. If the animal dies, the carcass should be burned or buried in a very deep pit, well covered with lime before filling with mud.

➤ *Haemorrhagic Septicaemia*: Hemorrhagic septicemia is a virulently infectious and contagious disease with a very high death rate. The infection can run through a herd of elephants very quickly, in about 10-15 days. Infection spreads by drinking infected water or eating contaminated food or inhaling infected droplets. Elephants, especially mature elephants, normally harbor pasturella organism in their body all the times without exhibiting clinical signs. Stress is often the precipitating factor that leads to full blown HS. Malnutrition, weakness, over-work, transportation and sudden change in diet or environmental conditions precipitate the disease. Elephants will die within 3-36 hours. HS in elephants is characterized by complete loss of appetite, frequent yawning, high fever, doughy and painful swelling of variable size in different parts of the body and contracted trunk. No treatment has proven to be effective in elephant HS.

> *Salmonellosis:* Salmonellosis of elephants is caused by *Salmonella javiana, S. weltervreden* and *S. typhimurium* and reported to be more fatal in baby elephants. Salmonellosis spread through infected food and water, especially food that has been stored a long time. Continuous watery diarrhea, poor appetite, exhaustion and fever are the clinical signs of salmonellosis. Separation of infected elephants, disinfection of the area, providing soft, easily digestible food such as ripe banana and antibiotic therapy are employed for the treatment and control of this disease.

> *Enterotoxemia*: Enterotoxaemia is caused by the toxin of *Clostridium perfringens* and toxin enters the gut through bacteria/toxin contaminated food. Affected elephant will be off feed, uncomfortable, restless and diarrhea leading to dehydration and death. Antitoxins and antibiotic therapy are indicated in enterotoxemia affected elephants.

Viral Diseases

➢ *Elephant Pox*: Elephant pox is a serious, infectious viral disease that has a history of being epidemic. Elephant pox is related to the human disease small pox. Asian elephants are more susceptible to pox virus infection than African elephants. Wild rodents are suspected of being the reservoir of elephant pox virus. The incidence of pox in elephants is comparatively rare. The important symptoms are edema of the head, trunk and lower abdomen, eruption of pustules on the buccal mucosa, tongue, ventral aspect of the trunk, ear flaps and abdomen. Severe conjunctivitis is a feature and it should be treated immediately with antibiotics otherwise vision will be affected due to opacity.

➢ *Foot and Mouth Disease*: FMD is an important contagious disease of hoofed livestock. FMD in elephants is caused by virus O type. The disease causing virus spreads through inhalation and contact with other infected animals. The symptoms noticed are vesicles/ulcers in the mouth, eruption and ulcers on the feet and febrile reaction. The body temperature may reach as high as 105 to 106 degree F. In extreme cases, complete longitudinal separation of the ventral skin of trunk may also be noticed. Limping is sometimes the first indicator of the disease. Affected animal should be separated from other elephants and fed with soft, highly nutritious and easily digestible food such as ripe banana.

➢ *Rabies*: Rabies is contracted by getting bitten by an infected animal. In elephants, rabies almost invariably brings paralysis and then death. The disease is characterized by listlessness, preference to stay in dark places, poor appetite, and failure to recognize the mahout, chasing and attacking humans and animals, unsteady gait, excessive salivation.

There is no effective treatment once the symptoms of rabies are seen. Prevention of rabies is a better choice. Proper bite wound treatment, separation of affected animal and securing the animals using chains is very necessary.

➢ *Herpes Virus Infection:* Herpes virus infection is usually found in elephants kept in confined enclosures with poor air circulation. Young animals are more susceptible. The clinical symptoms are not very obvious and laboratory diagnosis is the only method of diagnosis. Cyanosis is noticed in young elephants affecting tongue, mouth and inside the tip of the trunk. Disease signs become obvious when the immune status of animal is low.

➢ *Papilloma Warts*: Papilloma warts are not found very frequently in elephants. However, papilloma warts are most often seen in calves suffering from immunodeficiency. Warts are often found on the trunk and multiple warts can be seen. Multiple warts on the trunk can lead to irritation and animals will not be able to use its trunk properly. Many times, warts fall off on their own, but in few cases, treatment may be required. Warts can be removed by twisting them and then wart base is to be washed with disinfectant solution. This can be followed by topical application of antibacterial ointments.

Parasitic Diseases

➢ *Gastrointestinal helminthosis:* numerous species of helminths are commonly found, sometimes affecting 50% of the population in both wild and captive Indian elephants. Infected animals commonly show colic, foul smelling diarrhea, and gradually become anemic. In higher level of infection, mud eating, swelling on jowl, neck, brisket and abdomen are seen. Anthelmintic treatment is highly effective in treating gastrointestinal parasites in elephants.

➤ *Cutaneous filariasis:* Characterized by gooseberry size nodules on lateral and ventral side of the abdomen and hind limbs. Nodules rupture and exude blood intermittently. After some time bleeding stops and nodules get fibrosed. Microscopy of exudates can reveal microfilaria.

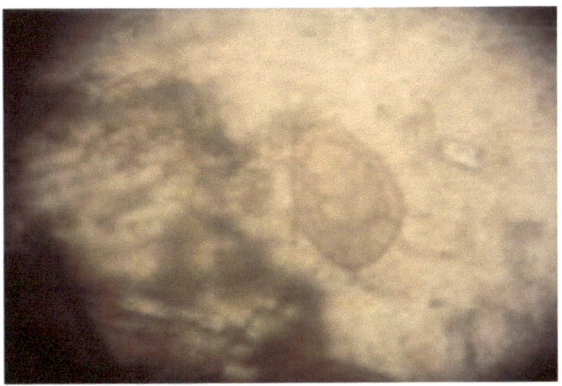

Figure 4: *Bivitellobilharzia nairi* detected in the feces of an apparently healthy female circus elephant. *Picture by Dr. Ravindra Bhoyar.*

➤ *Louse infestation:* It is common in both wild as well as captive elephants and infected animal becomes restless and gets pruritic lesions.

➤ *Trypanosomiasis:* Elephants exhibit intermittent fever, anorexia, swelling on dependent parts, anemia, and weakness. Extreme anemia and dehydration can easily lead to death.

➤ Most commonly found parasites in Indian elephants

Name of the parasite	Location
Round worms	
Amira pileata	Intestine
Bathmostomum sangeri	--
Cholangium epistomum	Intestine
Decrusia additicta	Intestine
Equinurbia sipunculiformis	Intestine

Grammocephalus varedatus	Liver
Indofilaria elephantis	Probably portal vessel
Indofilaria pattabhiramani	Cutaneous nodules
Murshidia falcifera	Intestine
Murshidia indica	Intestine
Murshidia murshida	Intestine
Parabronema indicum	Stomach
Parabronema smithi	Stomach
Quilonea renniei	Intestine
Quilonea travancra	Intestine
Amphistomes	
Pseudodiscus collinsi	Stomach & Intestine
Pseudodiscus hawkesi	Stomach & Intestine
Gastrodiscus secundus	Stomach & Intestine
Pfenderius papillatus	Stomach & Intestine
Blood fluke	
Bivitellobilharzia nairi	Portal vessels
Tapeworm	
Anoplocephala manubriata	Intestine
Protozoa	
Trypanosoma evansi	Blood
Louse	
Haematomyzus elephantis	Skin
Ticks	
Boophilus annulatus	Skin
Haemophysalis spinigera	Skin
Rhipicephalus haemophysaloides	Skin
Ornithodorus savignyi	Skin
Fly	
Cobboldia elephantis maggots	Stomach

Compiled from Healthcare Management of Captive Asian Elephants, Eds. Ajitkumar and others, Faculty of Veterinary and Animal Sciences, Kerala Agricultural University, Kerala 2009 and K.S. Subramania. Veterinary management of captive Asian elephants. Published by Tamil Nadu Veterinary and Animal Sciences University. 2010.

> *Gastric myiasis:* Elephants with gastric myasis exhibit diarrhea, dullness, colic and anorexia.

➢ *Tick infestation:* Not very common, due to less hair and regular bathing in captive elephants. However, wild elephants can have a small number of ticks.

Nonspecific diseases

➢ *Impaction of the colon:* Captive Asian elephants are very susceptible to impaction as feed intake is very high and movement is low. All parts of the colon or any one portion can get impacted with 50 to 100 kg of food materials which may be single or in multiple numbers. Elephants get impaction due to drinking large quantity of water after heavy work, due to improper food, low water intake or diseases of the teeth. Common symptoms seen are colic, straining, constipation, inappetite, which, if left unattended can progress to tympani, dehydration, vomiting, rupture of colon ultimately leading to death. Impaction can last up to 75 days; however the prognosis gets poorer with progression. Common line of treatment found suitable for Indian elephants is administration of analgesics and antispasmodics (Novalgin or Beralgan, 60-100 ml I/M), antihistamine (Avil 70-100 ml I/M), drugs acting on smooth muscles (Calcium pantothenate 50-70 ml, Perinorm 50-60 ml, Calcium borogluconate 450 to 900 ml I/V), antibiotics (Chloromycetin succinate 10-20gm or Ampicillin 10-15 gm I/V), parasymphathetic stimulants (Carbachol 5-10 mg or Prostigmin 3-4 mg I/M), electrolytes and dextrose saline, dextrose solution (15-25 liters I/V).

➢ *Foot rot:* foot rot has been observed in captive elephants due to the tethering of elephants for days together in unhygienic place. It can occur due stephanofilarial or fungal infections. The symptoms appear as black patches on foot space between and just above nails. The skin gets necrosed, sloughs off, leaving ulcers or granulating sponge like wounds that bleeds at the slightest pressure. Animals feel considerable pain and lameness. Commonly followed line of treatment includes cleaning the foot pad in 1/1000 with pot. permanganate solution, antiseptic foot bath in 1 to 2 per cent formalin or gentian violet, cauterization with copper sulfate, foot dressing with triple sulph mixed in 0l. Picis. liquidum, administration of streptomycin, and arsenicals.

➢ *Corneal opacity*:   Elephants get opacity due to vitamin A deficiency or injury. Discharge from the eyes, whitish patch or ulcer on the cornea and defective vision are the common symptoms noticed in affected elephants. Effective lines of treatment includes eye wash with normal saline or boric lotion, application with dionoresolvant cream, sub-conjuctival administration of Placentrex @ 2 ml on alternate days for three weeks, and vitamin A supplementation.

➢ *Arthritis*: elephants can get arthritis of any limb due to a contusion of joints on fall, hitting by logs, and ill treatment by the mahouts. Affected elephants show pain on movements, dragging of leg, swelling of joints, inability to bear body weight, tries to support body with trunk, and death in septicemic or suppurative arthritis. Commonly followed effective treatment involves I/M administration of analgesics like Novalgin 60 to 90 ml, anti-inflammatory drugs–Esgipyrin 60 to 90 ml, Artisone-S 90 ml, diuretics–Lasix 40 ml, antibiotics – Dicrysticin, 8 to 10 large doses or Ampicillin 10 to 15 gm or Crystalline penicillin 400 to 600 lakhs units, corticosteroids such as Betnesol 80 to 100 mg, Dexona or Hostacortin – H, oral administration of antirheumatic drugs, external application of counter irritants like iodine ointment or icthmol glycerine, exposure to infra red rays on the affected area.

> *Diseases Affecting Tusk:* Tusk is actually an incisor tooth and not a canine tooth as would be thought by many. The base of the tusks is embedded deeply in the elephant's skull, set in sockets under the eyes. Tusks are very strong and in a mature male elephant tusk grow at an average of about 17 cm a year.

Tusk diseases are of many kinds.

- *Cracked tusk:* Tusks may develop cracks as elephants habitually play with chains. The crack may be only near the tip or it may extend up to and into the base. In the latter case, the tissue that covers the base may be swollen. There will be copious watery discharge from the eyes if the tusk is infected. If the tusk is cracked or split near the tip, and if it is not severe, the condition may heal on its own if the elephant is taken off the work. If the crack is bad and severe, binding wire is tied round the tusk and periodically checked for infection. If the crack is of a chronic nature, tusk should be cleaned with clean water and disinfection solution. Antibiotic therapy and analgesic medication may be necessary in infected cases.

- *Decay of tusk (dental) pulp:* Accidental injuries, inappropriate trimming, and subsequent infections are the important causes of decay of pulp. Symptomatic treatment has to be followed.

- *Loose, wobbly tusks:* Loose and wobbly tusks are characterized by fowl smelling pus discharge from the base of the tusk. The elephant will regularly blow air or dirt on the area with its tusk. Washing the area with a solution of clean water and Povidone-iodine (1%) mixed in the ratio of 1:20 on a daily basis is warranted apart from antibiotic therapy.

- *Broken tusk:* Broken tusk is characterized by pus in the pulp cavity and the elephant will usually spray dirt with its trunk and use sticks to probe into the cavity.

In case of newly broken or cut tusks, bleeding is to be stopped and the cavity is to be cleaned with a disinfectant solution. The candle can be softened over a flame and can be inserted to block the cavity. In long standing and chronic cases all the dirt has to be washed, and the pus has to be cleaned out. Antibiotic therapy, analgesic and anti-inflammatory therapy is needed for fast and prompt recovery.

> *Diseases of Feet and Nails:* Elephant toenails are likely to break, split and fall off. Without treatment such conditions will damage the animal's general health. Poor nutrition and deficiency of minerals and certain vitamins can precipitate such conditions. Elephants working in slanted, hard or rocky surface are more affected with such problems.
>   o *Split toenails* are often found in elephants that most often walk in steep and hilly areas. Nail problems are particularly common in elephants. Split nails are characterized by elephant avoid putting weight on the foot and limping. Such elephants should be taken off the work. Nails should be filed across the split horizontal to the ground. File the bottom of the split down so it is smooth and does not cause the elephant to catch its foot and stumble. Otherwise crack will grow further.
>   o *Abnormal nail growth* is often found in elephants that must walk on steep and hilly terrain. Such elephants will not walk smoothly. Elephants may hobble. Resting the affected elephant, trimming any excess growth of nail and then file it smooth. Elephant's foot should be soaked in a diluted solution of copper sulfate. Treating foot and nail problems should be started very quickly and done correctly. Otherwise, the problem can compound itself and the elephant can become crippled or even die.

Table 6: Dose of commonly used pharmacologicals in elephants

Name of the drug	Major action	Dose	Route
Acepromazine	Sedation	50-60 mg/Ton	I.M.
Amino acid with sorbitol	Parenteral alimentation	100-200 ml/animal	I.V.
Ampicillin	Antibacterial	10-15 g/animal	I.V.
Analgin, Pitofenone,	Spasmolytic analgesic	60-90 ml	I.M.
Atropine	Anticholinergic	40-50 mg/Ton	I.M.
B-Complex	Vitamin	50 ml/animal	I.V.
Calcium borogluconate	Calcium	500-900 ml/animal	I.V.
Calcium pantothenate	Peristaltic	50-70 ml/animal	I.V.
Carbachol	Cholinergic	5-10 mg/animal	I.M.
Chloramphenicol succinate	Antibacterial	10-15 g	I.V.
Dexamethasone	Glucocorticoid	1-3 g/Ton	
Diprenorphine	Morphine antagonist	2 mg – 1 mg etorphine	I.M./I.V.
Doxapram	Analeptic	100 mg/Ton	I.M./I.V.
Ephedrine	Sympatho- mimetic	200-400 mg	I.M./I.V.
Etorphine	Sedative	1 mg/450 kg	I.M.
Frusemide	Diuretic	300-500 mg/animal	I.M.
Haloperidol	Sedative	40 mg/animal	PO/I.M.
Meperidine	Sedative	750-1500 mg/ Ton	I.M.
Metaclopramide	Antemetic	250-400 mg	I.V.
Morphine	Sedative	30-60 mg/Ton	I.M.
Morphine	Analgesic	60-200 mg/Ton with	I.M.

MADHUKAR DAMA & UPENDRA HA

Naloxone	Morphine antagonist	30-50 mg/animal	I.M./I.V.
Neostigmine	Cholinergic	4-5 mg/animal	I.M.
Oxygen		15-20 L/ min	
Penicillin	Antimicrobial	12-16 million. I. U	I.M.
Pheniramine	Antihistaminic	1700-2300 mg	I.M.
Phenylbutazone	Analgesic	10-15 g	I.M.
Xylazine	Sedative, Analgesic, Muscle relaxant,	80-150 mg/Ton	I.M.

Compiled from Healthcare Management of Captive Asian Elephants, Eds. Ajitkumar and others, Faculty of Veterinary and Animal Sciences, Kerala Agricultural University, Kerala 2009 and K.S. Subramania. Veterinary management of captive Asian elephants. Published by Tamil Nadu Veterinary and Animal Sciences University. 2010.

68

Table 7: Some common specific treatments in elephants

Drug	Dose	Route	Some trade names
Helminthosis			
Albendazole	2.5 mg/kg	Oral	Albomar
Bephenium hydroxy naphthoate	25 mg/kg	Oral	Alcopar
Fenbendazole	2-2.5 mg/kg	Oral	Panacur, Panfugal
Levamisole	2.5-3 mg/kg	Oral	Helmonil
Mebendazole	2.5-5 mg/kg	Oral	Eben, Mebex
Morantel citrate	2 mg/kg	Oral	Banminth Forte
Morantel tartarate	2-4 mg/kg	Oral	Banminth II
Oxibendazole	2.5 mg/kg	Oral	
Tetramisole	3-5 mg/kg	Oral	Nilverm, Curaminth
Thiabendazole	20 mg/kg	Oral	Thiabendal
Trypanosomiasis (Surra)			
Diminazene	3-8 mg/kg	I.M.	Berenil
Quinapyramine methyl sulphate	2-3 mg/kg	S.C.	Antricide
Tetanus			
Crystalline Penicillin	30-45 millium.I.U.	I.M./I.V.	
Antitetanus Serum	0.1-0.25 millium.I.U.	I.M.	
Diazepam	400-800 mg/ animal	I.M.	
Electrolyte Solution	15-25 liters	I.V.	
Filariasis			
Lithium Antimony	Filaricidal	60 ml/elephant/	Anthiomaline

69

thiomalate – solution		S.C.at tail fold	
Amphistomosis			
Hexachlorophene	10 mg/kg	Oral	Flukin
Rafoxanide	5-6 mg/kg	Oral	Ranide, Amfanide
Oxyclozanide	5-7.5 mg/kg	Oral	Distodin
Bivitellobilharziasis			
Lithium antimony thiomalate – 6%	200 ml/animal	S/C.	Antimosan, Anthiomaline
Cestodiasis			
Hexachlorophene	10 mg/kg	Oral	Flukin
Niclosamide	75-100 mg/kg	Oral	Niclex
Oxyclozanide	3-4 mg/kg	Oral	Distodin
Praziquantel	2.5-4 mg/kg	Oral	Droncit

Compiled from Healthcare Management of Captive Asian Elephants, Eds. Ajitkumar and others, Faculty of Veterinary and Animal Sciences, Kerala Agricultural University, Kerala 2009.

Chapter 5

PRACTICAL METHODS FOR FARMERS TO TACKLE ENTRY OF ELEPHANTS IN AGRICULTURE LANDS

Recent times have witnessed an increase in the straying of elephants in human habitats as well as cultivated lands. This results in loss of crops, damages to the property, and in some unfortunate cases loss of lives. Though there is compensation for affected persons for their losses, loss of life cannot be compensated by any means. Hence, farmers living near to elephant habitats should take measures to prevent the entry of elephants in their areas. However, the measures should be safe and practical, with no chances of causing lethal damages to elephants, as elephants are a precious natural assets and integral part of our cultural and religious heritage. Any, or combination of the following methods can be practiced by farmers to prevent the elephant related damages.

1. Crops such as chilly, tobacco, capsicum, tea and oil seeds can be grown on the boundary of fields as these are distasteful to elephants.
2. Try to avoid the plantation of crops favored by elephants such as jackfruit, banana, and coconut on the forest side.
3. Do not plant crops on an area of 5 meter (buffer zone) around the fields to increase the sighting of elephants.
4. Carbide cannon can be fired in the air to make a loud noise to scare the elephants.
5. String of cowbells, empty tins and paper ribbons can be tied along the fence to detect the entry of elephants.
6. Wood can be burnt all night to sight elephants. If available, Chinese Bamboo can be burnt in this fire to make regular sounds as cavities inside blast.
7. Firecrackers can be thrown towards elephants to scare them away.

8. During elephant raiding seasons, all night patrol would increase the chances of sighting elephants before they enter the fields.
9. Bricks prepared by elephant dung and ground chillies can be burnt all night to maintain noxious smoke that keeps elephants away.
10. Trip alarm system, which goes on as elephants step on, can be mounted on the boundary of the field to detect the arrival of elephants.
11. Farmers can build one watchtower every half kilometre to sight the arriving elephants.
12. Farmers can blow whistles to alert neighboring farmers on sighting elephants.
13. Whips made of bark can be used to make loud noise similar to gunshot to scare the elephants.
14. A powerful and novel method is tying ropes to the bee boxes fixed along the boundary of field. As elephants enter, the ropes will be automatically shaken, exposing the elephants to noxious stings. This is one of the most effective methods to scare away the elephant for a very long time, in addition to generation of income from honey.
15. Capsicum oleoresin repellent can be sprayed towards approaching elephants to deter them immediately as it causes noxious irritation and burning sensation.
16. Ropes made from chilli can be tied along the fences to deter elephants. Further, chilli oil applied on fences also effectively deters elephants.
17. Farmers have to work in collaboration with neighboring farmers to rotate patrolling duties and alert each other on sighting elephants.

Farmers must try to shift from one method to other every year, as elephants get used to empty threats. Also note that these are temporary methods, and farmers can go for permanent methods like solar fencing, which is very costly, once these methods fail

Chapter -6

LEGAL ASPECTS OF INDIAN ELEPHANTS

➢ In addition to the laws governing the rights of an animal, elephants have numerous special rights because of its cultural, ecological, and economical significance.

➢ After inclusion of elephants in the schedule-I of the Wildlife Protection Act – 1972, elephants gained a highest degree of legal protection in India.

➢ Hunting or capturing of elephants is banned; however, capture or killing of rogue elephant, capture for scientific studies, and capture for zoological parks or population control is allowed with prior permission of the government.

➢ Commercial trade of elephant as well as parts derived from elephants is prohibited.

➢ Domesticated elephants are also having protection similar to the wild elephants.

➢ No person can keep, possess or acquire an elephant without an ownership certificate issued by the chief wildlife warden or any other authorized officer.

➢ Only the persons possessing an ownership certificate can transfer elephants by way of sale, gift or otherwise.

➢ A person, having an ownership certificate, is required to inform the concerned chief wildlife warden within 30 days in case of transfer of elephant to another state.

➢ The domesticated elephant is excluded from the definition of livestock. However, the Act recognizes a domesticated elephant as a 'vehicle' to facilitate its confiscation if used for committing any offense.

➢ The zoos recognized by the Central Zoo Authority are exempted from possessing ownership certificates. Zoos are also required to follow standards and norms prescribed under the Recognition of Zoos Rules, 1992 for keeping elephants in captivity.

- Offenses relating to elephants under the WPA-1972 cannot be compounded.
- For general offenses concerning elephants, the offender can be punished with imprisonment from one year to six years and a fine not less than Rs.5000.
- For offenses relating to illegal trade in elephants and ivory, offender can be imprisoned for up to 7 years.
- Any elephant captured or kept in violation of the WPA-1972 is a government property and liable for confiscation.
- Import and export of elephants are governed by the Import-Export Policy of the Ministry of Commerce.
- Zoological parks recognized scientific institutes, circus companies and private individuals can import elephants subject to the recommendation of the chief wildlife warden and the provisions of the Convention on International Trade in Endangered Species of Wild Fauna and Flora (CITES).
- Export of elephants is prohibited, except for non-commercial export for scientific, zoological or educational purposes, subject to the recommendation of the Ministry of Environment and Forests.
- Violation of the Import-Export Policy is an offense under the Customs Act, 1962.

The domesticated elephants are also subject to the provisions of the Prevention of Cruelty to Animals Act, 1960 (PCA-1960) and the various rules framed thereunder, viz. The Prevention of Cruelty to Draught and Pack Animals Rules, 1965, the Performing Animals Rules, 1973 and the Prevention of Cruelty (Capturing of Animals) Rules, 1972. "Cruelty" has not been defined in the Act. However, certain acts of omissions and commissions described in the Act constitute cruelty punishable under the Act. Some of the activities recognized as cruelty include: subjecting an elephant to beating, over-riding, over-loading, torturing, willful and unreasonable administration of any injurious substance, confinement to a cage which does not permit it a reasonable opportunity of movement, conveying or carrying in such a manner as to subject it to unnecessary suffering, inciting to fight any other animal for the purpose of entertainment, depriving an elephant of sufficient food, water or shelter.

The rules under the PCA-1960 prohibit use of elephants for drawing any vehicle or carrying any load for more than nine hours a day; use of any spiked stick or sharp equipment for driving or riding an elephant; and capture of animals except by 'sack and loop' method, tranquilizing guns or any other method which renders the animals insensible to pain before capture. The rules stipulate registration of trainers and exhibitors of performing elephants.

PROJECT ELEPHANT

Project Elephant (PE), a centrally sponsored scheme, was launched in February 1992 to provide financial and technical support to major elephant bearing States in the country for the protection of elephants, their habitats and corridors. It also seeks to address the issues of human-elephant conflict and welfare of domesticated elephants.

The Project is being implemented in 13 States / UTs, viz. Andhra Pradesh , Arunachal Pradesh, Assam, Jharkhand , Karnataka , Kerala , Meghalaya , Nagaland , Orissa , Tamil Nadu , Uttranchal , Uttar Pradesh and West Bengal.

Based on the proposals received in the form of Annual Plan of Operations, Government of India provides financial and technical assistance to State/UT Governments for wildlife protection under the various Centrally Sponsored Schemes – *Development of National Parks and Sanctuaries, Project Tiger* and *Project Elephant*. The State-wise details of funds which have been released under this project are given below (RS in lakhs):

S.No.	State	2002-03	2003-04	2004-05	2005-06	2006-07*
1	Andhra Pradesh	50	55	48	60	40
2	Arunachal Pradesh	52	61	59	71.5	45
3	Assam	116	134.1	130	40	120
4	Jharkhand	45	93	105.96	75	90
5	Karnataka	93	149.66	186.22	168	110
6	Kerala	111.88	188.28	167.4	170	100
7	Meghalaya	41	64	70	30	-

8	Nagaland	49	42	29	48	20
9	Orissa	108.39	116.1	137.96	114	100
10	Tamil Nadu	71.26	117	84	112	80
11	Uttranchal	107	129	138.9	82	71.86
12	West Bengal	86.47	119.95	148.54	181	120
13	Tripura	3	16	17	0	-
14	Mizoram	5	-	0	0	-
15	Uttar Pradesh	-	-	12	0	40
	TOTAL	939	1285.09	1333.98	1151.5	975.00**

*The sum indicates the funds released till August 2007. ** This includes Rs. 40.56 (lakhs) released to Maharashtra*

Source: *Project Elephant.*

There are only 17 states in which elephants exist in the wild state. Project Elephant has declared 24 elephant reserves in 12 states to protect elephant populations in the wild and develop their habitat. It was launched in the year 1991-92 as a sequel to a series of efforts to conserve this magnificent species covering primarily twelve states of India, namely Assam, Arunachal Pradesh, Bihar, Andhra Pradesh, Karnataka, Kerala, Meghalaya, Nagaland, Orissa, Tamil Nadu, Uttar Pradesh and West Bengal.

Animal Habitats in India (Sq km)		
North -East Region	**Maximum Area**	**Minimum Area**
State		
Arunachal Pradesh	7800	7000
Assam	20000	17000
Meghalaya	10000	9000
Nagaland	13000	1000
Mizoram	600	400
Manipur	350	250
Tripura	1500	1000
West Bengal (North)	2800	2300
Total for North East Region	**44350**	**37950**
Eastern Part of the Country		
West Bengal (South)	1800	1500

Jharkhand	8500	7500
Bihar	500	300
Orissa	15000	12000
Total for East	**25800**	**21300**
North- West Part of The Country		
Uttaranchal	4500	4000
Uttar Pradesh	1000	500
Total for North-West	**5500**	**4500**
Southern Part of the Country		
Karnataka	20000	17000
Kerala	9500	9000
Andhra Pradesh	1300	800
Total of South	**42800**	**36800**
Islands		
Andaman & Nicobar	600	300
Grand Total	**119550**	**101350**

Source: Project Elephant.

Activities of Project Elephant

- ➢ Various activities are being carried out under this project.
- ➢ Existing natural habitats and migratory routes of elephants are restored ecologically.
- ➢ Scientific and planned management are being developed for conservation of elephant habitats and viable population of wild Asiatic elephants in India to reduce man-elephant conflict in crucial habitats.
- ➢ Promotional measures have been applied.
- ➢ Domestic stock activities in crucial elephant habitats have been stopped.
- ➢ Wild elephants give protection against poachers and also against an unnatural cause of deaths.

➢ Research on Elephant management related issues.
➢ Public education and awareness programs and Eco-development are other measures under implementation.

Census in Elephant Reserves in India (2005)

➢ The first time an exclusive exercise for enumeration of wild elephants in the ERs was done during Feb-May 2005.
➢ This exercise also sought to experiment with two sampling methods, viz. Block Sampling; and Line Transact-Dung Count (with Retrospective Method of Calculating Dung Decay Rate).
➢ Project Elephant arranged Training of Trainers and also issued detailed guidelines to the Chief Wild Life Wardens (CWLWs) and the Field Coordinators.

Monitoring of Illegal Killing of Elephants (Mike) sites:

➢ Project Elephant has been formally implementing MIKE (Monitoring of Illegal Killing of Elephants) programme of CITES in 10 ERs since 01.04.2004.
➢ These include Shiwalik (Uttaranchal); Eastern Dooars (West Bengal); Mayurbhanj (Orissa); Ripu-Chirang and Dehing-Patkai (Assam); Garo Hills (Meghalaya); Deomali (Arunchal Pradesh); Wayanad (Kerala), Mysore (Karnataka) and Nilgiri (Tamil Nadu).

Research, consultancy and training projects:

➢ Project elephant conducted a 36-months research project (2003-04 to 2006-07) with the help of the Central Rice Research Institute (CRRI), Cuttack, for developing high yielding varieties of paddy not relished by elephants; developing elephant-proof storage bins for food grains; and developing elephant repellents.
➢ Project elephant has also completed two projects each of 36 months duration (2003-04 to 2006-07) with the help of the Assam Agricultural University on 'Disease Management in Captive Elephants' and 'Anatomical Studies on the Asian Elephant'.

➤ The Wildlife Institute of India (WII) studied the impact of the relocation of the Gujjars on the flora and fauna of Rajaji National Park during (2004-05 to 2005-06) in a small project assigned by Project Elephant.

➤ The Indian Statistical Institute, Kolkata completed a small consultancy project to help the West Bengal Forest Department in carrying out a sample-based enumeration of elephants during 2005 which was assigned by the PE.

➤ Project Elephant has been organizing regular refresher courses for veterinarians dealing with wild and domesticated elephants at Kerala Agricultural University, Trichur and Assam Agricultural University, Guwahati.

Chapter-7

OVERVIEW OF POST-MORTEM OF ELEPHANT

> All the principles pertinent to necropsy of a livestock apply to the necropsy of elephants also. In addition, special considerations are taken keeping in view that elephant is a wild animal, that some wild animal diseases are notifiable and the elephant has special anatomical features.

> A proper permission should be obtained from concerned authority as elephants are protected under schedule I of wildlife (Protection) act 1972.

> Post-mortem should be conducted under daylight.

> All the observations should be duly noted down.

> Anthrax and tuberculosis are reported in elephants, which necessitates the use of protective clothing during the necropsy procedure.

> Carcass suspected of anthrax should be subjected to blood smear examination before opening the body.

> Malicious poisoning should be suspected in mysteriously dead elephants.

> Approximation of the time of death can be done by observing

  o Hypostatic congestion (lividity): due to large size elephants frequently show livid patches in the subcutis on the side touching the ground.

  o Rigor mortis: this may set with death or take up to 24 hours or longer. On average, rigor mortis sets in 1-4 hours and lasts up to 17 hours. Rigor mortis is less pronounced in weak animals and sets early.

  o Decomposition: depending on the condition of the animal and the surroundings, decomposition begins in 6 to 36 hours. Wild elephant carcasses are commonly found in decomposed condition.

Equipment set

1. Six large necropsy knives and knife sharpener
2. Sterile sample collection set. Include vials, labels, slides, bottles, waterproof marking pens, gloves, etc.
3. 10% neutral buffered formalin (about 7 liters)
4. Field acid-fast staining kit (to determine the presence or absence of *Mycobacterium Sp.*)
5. Gluteraldehyde, 2.5-4% (at least 100mls)
6. Scale for obtaining organ weights.
7. Tape measure (metric), at least 2 meters long.
8. Small and large Chain saw, axe and hacksaw.
9. Hammers, chisels and handsaws.
10. Six small hand meat hooks
11. Hoist/crane/small tractor
12. Heavy straps, chains, ropes
13. Carts on rollers to move heavy parts.
14. Coveralls, boots, gloves, caps, masks, protective eye and head gear, face shields
15. Accessible water supply with hose.
16. Camera and size reference (ruler)
17. First aid kit.
18. Surgical masks approved for TB exposure
19. Biohazard bag (red bags)
20. Leak proof Styrofoam boxes or other leak proof boxes
21. Disinfectant solution (tuberculo-cidal)
22. Handsaws
23. Bone cutter
24. Crow-bar
25. Scalpel handles
26. Scalpel blades
27. Surgical scissors
28. Forceps
29. Chisel

30. Iron spatula
31. Ropes
32. Magnifying glass
33. Torches (Flash light)
34. Emergency lamps/Generator
35. A vehicle fitted with light focusing facilities.
36. Metal detector (to search bullets)

Pre-post-mortem observations

Following points has to be noted down

> Place or geographical location where carcass was discovered
> Current weather conditions - drought, flood, storm, and ambient temperature.
> Common name, zoological name, sex, approximate age and number of animals died.
> History of the case should include duration and severity of illness if any, morbidity, nutritional condition, symptoms before death, other deaths, treatments and any other specific observations.
> Approximate weight and age of the elephant.
> Mode of transportation of the carcass with date and time of death if known.
> Signs of struggle or other evidence relating to the death.
> Wounds, signs of predation, presence of external parasites (ticks, mites, fleas, etc.), fracture, broken or missing teeth, horns, tusk, bruise, bleeding etc.

Post-mortem procedure

> Position the elephant on back with left side up to facilitate observation of the cecum and colon
> Decapitate, open the cranium and remove the brain
> Cut the vertebrae and examine spinal cord.
> Examine the eyes and collect one eye for histopathology
> Examine the ears.
> Examine the legs and remove them intact

➢ Examine the nails and sole for lesions.

➢ Incise the skin mid-ventrally, avoiding mammary gland in females, to expose the sternum.

➢ Examine mammary lymph node

➢ Extend the incision to the perineal region, working around the external genitalia in males, and examine the penis and prepuce.

➢ Expose thoracic cavity by cutting ribs at the costochondral junction, and examine the contents by separating pleural attachments.

➢ Take out the heart, lungs and diaphragm intact.

➢ Incise pericardium and examine for thickening and increased abnormal contents of pericardial sac.

➢ Cut open the heart on the right side first and then left side, examine the muscle, endocardium, valves and also major vessels.

➢ Examine the lung by palpation and incision for lumps and nodules.

➢ Examine the mediastinal lymph nodes.

➢ Open the abdominal cavity and examine the viscera in-situ for the presence of fluid, water, adhesion and displacement of organs.

➢ Open the pelvic cavity by cutting the pubis and examine the organs.

➢ Examine the mouth, tongue, tonsil, nasal cavity, trunk, nasal passage, intercommunicating nasal canals for lesions.

➢ Remove the tongue, larynx, trachea and esophagus by cutting soft tissues and the mandible.

➢ Examine the thyroid and parathyroid glands.

➢ Expose the esophagus, larynx, and trachea and examine bronchial lymph node.

➢ Examine and remove the omentum, spleen, pancreas and the samples.

➢ Examine the stomach and its contents.

➢ Examine the liver for lesions.

➢ Straighten the intestine and cut open and examine the contents.

➢ Collect gastrointestinal content specimens for toxicology and tissue samples for histopathology

➢ Examine the cecum and colon.

➢ Free the liver from the attachment. Examine the surface and cut surface for lesions

➢ Measure the length of the tusks and the circumference at the base on either side.

- ➢ Examine the adrenals, kidneys and ureter
- ➢ Remove the kidneys from its capsule and incise it longitudinally and examine the cortex, medulla and pelvis.
- ➢ Expose the urinary bladder and examine its contents.
- ➢ Open and examine the uterus, vagina and vulva.
- ➢ Locate testes in the sub lumbar area, incise and examine the cut surface.
- ➢ Examine testes and accessory sex glands.
- ➢ Examine bone and skeletal muscles, especially shoulder and thigh muscle for lesions
- ➢ Dissect sciatic nerve and collect samples.
- ➢ Remove a long bone and collect the bone marrow.
- ➢ Examine the umbilicus in young calves.
- ➢ Examine the joints for erosions on articular surface.
- ➢ Examine the skin for lesion and collect full thickness of abdominal skin.
- ➢ Examine temporal glands.

Model post-mortem report

Institution /Owner:
Address:
Post-mortem No.:
Species:
Age:
Sex:
Color:
Wild:
Wild caught:
Captive born:
Date and time of death:
Death location:
Necropsy date:
Time:
Necropsy location:
Clinical history, circumstantial history and tentative clinical diagnosis:
Blood smear examination:
General findings:
Body cavities and sinuses:
Respiratory system:
Cardiovascular system:
Digestive system:
Spleen:
Urinary system:
Reproductive system:
Musculoskeletal system:
Central nervous system:
Endocrine system:
Any other general findings:
Results of Special laboratory tests:
Summary Post-mortem diagnosis: Etiopathological diagnosis (based on observations and laboratory results):
Post-mortem examiner: Date: Signature:

Modified and Adapted from Jacob V. Cheeran and N. Diwakaran Nair. Techniques & procedure for post-mortem of elephants. A Handbook for Veterinarians, Biologists & Elephant Managers. Published by Project Elephant and Central Zoo Authority, Ministry of Environment and Forests New Delhi. First Edition 2003.

REFERENCES AND FURTHER READING

1. Ajithkumar Santra. Handbook on wild and zoo animals. International book distributing company. 2008.
2. Chaleamchat Somgird, Tulyawat Sutthipat and Waroot Wongkalasin. General healthcare in captive elephants. Elephant Research and Education Center.
3. Chaleamchat Somgird. Anatomy and Physiology. Elephant Research and Education Center.
4. Chatchote Thitaram. Breeding management of Asian elephants. Elephant Research and Education Center.
5. Healthcare Management of Captive Asian Elephants, Eds. Ajitkumar and others, Faculty of Veterinary and Animal Sciences, Kerala Agricultural University, Kerala 2009.
6. IUCN. The Asian Elephant.
7. Jacob V. Cheeran and N. Diwakaran Nair. Techniques & procedure for post-mortem of elephants. A Handbook for Veterinarians, Biologists & Elephant Managers. Published by Project Elephant and Central Zoo Authority, Ministry of Environment and Forests New Delhi. First Edition 2003.
8. K.S. Subramania. Veterinary management of captive Asian elephants. Published by Tamil Nadu Veterinary and Animal Sciences University. 2010.
9. Murray E Fowler; R Eric Miller. Zoo and wild animal medicine : current therapy. St. Louis, MO : Saunders/Elsevier, 2008.
10. Murray E Fowler; Susan K Mikota. Biology, medicine, and surgery of elephants. Ames, Iowa: Blackwell Pub., 2006.
11. Preecha Phuangkum, Richard C. Lair and Taweepoke Angkawanith. Elephant care manual for mahouts and camp managers. Forest industry organization, Ministry of natural resources and environment, Food and agriculture organization of the united nations, Regional office for asia and the pacific Bangkok, 2005.
12. Various websites and internet books freely available online

Wildlife of India. Project Elephant.
Source: http://pib.nic.in/release/release.asp?relid=39691.